Scoping review of the effectiveness of mental health services

Ruth Jepson
Zelda Di Blasi
Kath Wright
Gerben Ter Riet*

NHS Centre for Reviews and Dissemination
University of York
York
Y01 5DD

Tel: 01904 433635
Fax: 01904 433661

*Also affiliated to:
Dept of Epidemiology
Maastricht University
6200 MD Maastricht
The Netherlands

March 2001

Commissioning Support Unit

© 2001 NHS Centre for Reviews and Dissemination, University of York

ISBN 1 900640 19 8

This report can be ordered from: Publications Office, NHS Centre for Reviews and Dissemination, University of York, York YO10 5DD. Telephone 01904 433648; Facsimile: 01904 433661: email: crdpub@york.ac.uk
Price £12.50

The NHS Centre for Reviews and Dissemination is funded by the NHS Executive and the Health Departments of Wales and Northern Ireland. The views expressed in this publication are those of the authors and not necessarily those of the NHS Executive or the Health Departments of Wales or Northern Ireland.

Printed by York Publishing Services Ltd.

ACKNOWLEDGEMENTS

The authors wishes to thank the Department of Health for providing the funding for this review, and Jos Kleijnen, Director at NHS CRD for his comments and support. The CRD team also wishes to thank Sarah Byford, research fellow at the Centre of Health Economics at York, for her assistance in part 2 of the review.

ADVISORY BOARD

Jennifer Beecham
PSSRU, Kent
The University
Canterbury
Kent
CT2 7NF

Simon Gilbody
NHS CRD
University of York
York
YO1 5DD

Gary Hogman
National Schizophrenia Fellowship
30 Tabernacle Street
London
EC2A 4DD

Peter Kennedy
Director
Northern Centre for Mental Health
Durham

Martin Knapp
Centre for the Economics of Mental Health
Institute of Psychiatry
De Crespigny Park
London SE5 8AF

Juliet Koprowska
SPSW
University of York
York
YO1 5DD

Katie Needham
Health Studies
University of York
York
YO1 5DD

Graham Thornicroft
Professor of Community Psychiatry
Institute of Psychiatry Kings College
London

Director of R&D South London And
Maudsley NHS Trust

Head of Health Services Research
Dept IOP KCL

Paula Whitty
Consultant/Senior Lecturer in Medical Care Epidemiology
Newcastle City Health Trust
Milvain Building
Newcastle General Hospital
Westage Road
Newcastle upon Tyne
NE4 6BE

Mark Whyte
Health Studies
University of York
York
YO1 5DD

NHS CENTRE FOR REVIEWS AND DISSEMINATION

The NHS Centre for Reviews and Dissemination (CRD) is a facility commissioned by the NHS Research and Development Division. Its aim is to identify and review the results of good quality health research and to disseminate actively the findings to key decision makers in the NHS and to consumers of health care services. In this way health care professionals and managers can ensure their practice reflects the best available research evidence. The reviews will cover: the effectiveness of care for particular conditions; the effectiveness of health technologies; and evidence on efficient methods of organising and delivering particular types of health care.

Further Information

General Enquiries:	01904 433634
Information Service	01904 433707
Publications:	01904 433648
Fax:	01904 433661
Email:	revdis@york.ac.uk

CRD Reports

1.	Which Way Forward for the Care of Critically Ill Children? (1995)	£7.50
4.	Undertaking Systematic Reviews of Research on Effectiveness. CRD's Guidance for those Carrying Out or Commissioning Reviews (2nd edition 2001)	£12.50
5.	Ethnicity and Health (1996)	£12.50
6.	Making Cost-Effectiveness Information Accessible: The NHS Economic Evaluation Database Project. (CRD Guidance for Reporting Critical Summaries of economic evaluations (1996)	£6.00
7.	A Pilot Study of 'Informed Choice' Leaflets on Positions in Labour (1996)	£7.50
8.	Concentration and Choice in the Provision of Hospital Services (1997)	
	Summary Report	£6.00
	Part I - Hospital Volume and Quality of Health Outcomes	£12.50
	Part II - Volume and the scope of activity and hospital costs	£9.50
	Part III - Concentration, patient accessibility and utilisation of services	£7.50
	Complete set of reports	£30.00
9.	Preschool Vision Screening: Results of a Systematic Review (1997)	£9.50
10.	Systematic Review of Interventions in the Treatment and Prevention of Obesity (1997)	£12.50 £12.50
11.	A Systematic Review of the Effectiveness of Interventions for Managing Childhood Nocturnal Enuresis (1997)	£12.50
13.	Screening for Ovarian Cancer: A Systematic Review (1998)	£12.50
14.	Women and Secure Psychiatric Services: A Literature Review (1999)	£12.50
15.	Systematic Review of the international literature on the epidemiology Of mentally disordered offenders (1999)	£12.50
16.	Scoping Review of Literature on the Health and Care of Mentally Disordered Offenders (1999)	£12.50
17.	Therapeutic Community Effectiveness: Community Treatment for People with Personality Disorders and Mentally Disordered Offenders (1999)	£12.50
18.	A Systematic Review of Water Fluoridation (2000)	£20.00
19.	The Longevity of Dental Restorations: A Systematic Review (2001)	£20.00
20.	Informed Choice in Maternity Care: An Evaluation of Evidence Based Leaflets (2001)	£20.00

TABLE OF CONTENTS

Glossary	vi
Executive summary	ix
Background and rationale for the review	1
Remit of the report	2
PART 1. SCOPING REVIEW OF MENTAL HEALTH DELIVERY INTERVENTIONS	3
Aims	3
Objectives	3
Methods	3
Search Strategy	4
Applying inclusion/exclusion criteria and data extraction	4
Results	5
Quality of included reviews	5
1. NSF standard one: mental health promotion	6
2. NSF standards two and three: primary care and access to services	7
3. NSF standards four and five: effective services for people with sever mental illness	10
4. NSF standard six: caring about carers	18
5. NSF standard seven: preventing suicide	20
Discussion	24
Conclusions	26
PART 2. COST-EFFECTIVENESS OF MENTAL HEALTH SERVICE DELIVERY INTERVENTIONS	28
Background	28
Aim	28
Objectives	28
Inclusion criteria	28
Search strategy	29
Results	29
1. NSF standard one: mental health promotion	29
2. NSF standards two and three: primary care and access to services	29
3. NSF standards four and five: effective services for people with severe mental illness	32
4. NSF standard 6: caring for carers	34
5. NSF standard 7: preventing suicide	34
Discussion	34
Limitations of present review	35
References	36
Appendix 1. Search strategy for identifying systematic reviews of mental health service delivery interventions	40
Appendix 2. Criteria for assessing quality of reviews of effectiveness (DARE inclusion criteria)	46
Appendix 3. Data extraction tables for systematic reviews of health service delivery interventions	47
Appendix 4. Scoping 24-hour mental health services	91
Appendix 5. Search strategy for identifying economic evaluations of mental health service delivery interventions	96
Appendix 6. Data extraction tables for cost-effectiveness papers	99

GLOSSARY

Assertive outreach (assertive community treatment, intensive case management)[1]
An active form of treatment delivery: the service can be taken to the service users rather than expecting them to attend for treatment. Care and support may be offered in the service user's home or some other community setting, at times suited to the service user rather than focused on service providers' convenience. Workers are likely to be involved in direct delivery of practical support, care co-ordination and advocacy as well as more traditional therapeutic input. Closer, more trusting relationships may be developed with the aim of maintaining service users in contact with the service and complying with effective treatments.

Care co-ordinator (or key worker)[1]
A worker (team member) with responsibility for co-ordinating CPA reviews for mental health service users with complex needs and for communicating with others involved in the service user's care. Care co-ordinators usually have the most contact with the service user.

Care management[1]
See case management

Care programme approach (CPA)[1]
The CPA provides a framework for care co-ordination of service users under specialist mental health services. The main elements are a care co-ordinator, a written care plan, and at higher levels, regular reviews by the multi-disciplinary health team and integration with the social services care management system. Updated and simplified guidelines, with two levels of CPA, standard and enhanced, will be published by the Department of Health in association with the National Service Framework.

Carers[1]
Relatives or friends who voluntarily look after individuals who are sick, disabled, vulnerable or frail.

Case management (in the UK called care management)[2]
In its simplest form (referred to as 'brokerage') case management is a means of co-ordinating services. Each mentally ill person is assigned a 'case manager' who is expected to:
(i) assess that person's needs;
(ii) develop a care plan;
(iii) arrange for suitable care to be provided;
(iv) monitor the quality of the care provided; and,
(v) maintain contact with the person[26].

'Brokerage' case managers often lack clinical qualifications and tend to work outside established psychiatric services. In the UK, the model adopted for care management is that of 'extended brokerage' case management.[3]

Cochrane Protocol
A protocol for a Cochrane systematic review should describe the rationale for the review; the objectives; and the methods that will be used to locate, select and critically appraise studies, and to collect and analyse data from the included studies.

Cochrane Review
A Cochrane Review is a systematic, up-to-date summary of reliable evidence of the benefits and risks of healthcare. Cochrane Reviews are intended to help people make practical decisions. Reviewers adhere to guidelines published in the Cochrane Handbook, are published on The Cochrane Library and are updated regularly.

Community mental health nurse[1]
Mental health nurse with specific expertise in working with patients in the community, in functioning in a multi-disciplinary team and in working across the inpatient/community interface.

Community mental health team[1]
A multi-disciplinary team offering specialist assessment, treatment and care to people in their own homes and the community. The team should involve nursing, psychiatric, social work, clinical psychology and occupational therapy membership, with ready access to other therapies and expertise, for example specialist psychotherapy, art therapy, and pharmacy. Adequate administrative and information technology (IT) support is vital.

Cost-benefit analysis[4]
Cost-benefit analysis (CBA) measures both costs and benefits in monetary values and calculates net monetary gains or losses (presented as a cost-benefit ratio).

Cost-effectiveness analysis[4]
A cost-effectiveness analysis (CEA) compares interventions with a common outcome (such as blood pressure level) to discover which produces the maximum outcome for the same input of resources in a given population.

Cost-utility analysis[4]
A cost-utility analysis (CUA) measures the benefits of alternative treatments or types of care by using utility measures such as Quality-adjusted Life Years (QALYs) and may present relative costs per QALY.

Day care in the community
Types of day care include: acute day care; transitional day care; therapeutic day care; long-term supportive day care; generic day care.

Economic evaluation[4]
Full economic evaluations are studies in which a comparison of two or more treatments or care alternatives is undertaken and in which both the costs and outcomes of the alternatives are examined. Full economic evaluations in the scope of the NHS Economic Evaluation Database are regarded as cost-benefit analyses, cost-utility analyses, and cost-effectiveness analyses (see glossary entries for a full definition of these terms). Cost-minimisation analyses and cost-consequence analyses are also included.

First-level advice from *NHS Direct*[1]
First-level advice is to provide comprehensive information about services and treatments that are available locally. If necessary, NHS Direct will aim to ensure callers are directed to the right service, providing referral on to specialist helplines or mental health services.

Home treatment[1]
Treatment may be offered in a patient's home rather than in clinical settings, either by a separate team or by a community mental health team. Frequent home visits by various members of the multi-disciplinary team can lead to an avoidance of some hospital admissions and provide support to informal carers. Such services should be available at weekends and in evenings as well as during office hours.

Mental disorder[1]
Mental disorder is defined in the 1983 Mental Health Act as 'mental illness, arrested or incomplete development of mind, psychopathic disorder and any other disorder or disability of mind'. The Act does not define mental illness, which is a matter for clinical judgement.

Mental health[1]
An individual's ability to manage and cope with the stresses and challenges of life.

Mental health organisations[1]
Health and social care commissioners and providers of specialist mental health care, including independent sector providers.

Mental Health Promotion
Mental health promotion could include any activity that actively fosters good mental health through increasing health promoting factors and decreasing factors that damage or reduce mental health for both individuals and communities.

Mental health services[1]
Specialist provision of mental health and social care provision integrated across organisational boundaries.

Mental illness[1]
Range of diagnosable mental disorders that excludes learning disability and personality disorder.

Primary care groups[1]
Groups of family doctors and community nurses with resources for commissioning healthcare. Their budget is based on their local population's share of available resources for hospital and community health services, the general medical services cash-limited budget, and prescribing.

Risk assessment
Prediction of likelihood that an individual will commit violence directed to self or others. Refers to diagnostic/predictive instruments

Service user/s[1]
People who need health and social care for their mental health problems. They may be individuals who live in their own homes, are staying in care, or are being cared for in hospital.

Severe mental illness[1]
Severe mental illness was defined by the NSF working group in as follows:

- there must be a mental disorder as designated by a mental health professional (psychiatrist, mental health nurse, clinical psychologist, occupational therapist or mental health social worker) **and either**
- there must have been a score of 4 (very severe problem) on at least one, or a score of 3 (moderately severe problem) on at least two, of the Health of Nations Outcome Scale (HoNOS) items 1-10 (excluding item 5 'physical illness or disability problems') during the previous six months **or**
- there must have been a significant level of service usage over the past five years as shown by:
- a total of six months in a psychiatric ward/ day hospital, or three admissions to hospital *or*
- day hospital/ six months of psychiatric community care involving more than one worker *or*
- the perceived need for such care if unavailable or refused.

Social care[1]
Personal care for vulnerable people, including individuals with special needs which stem from their age or physical or mental disability, and children who need care and protection. Examples of social care services are residential care homes, home helps and home care services. Local authorities have statutory responsibilities for providing social care.

Supported accommodation in the community
Two types of supported accommodation. Firstly, dedicated supported housing schemes and tenancies with outreach support schemes. These schemes involve having self-contained apartments located in one building or site, specifically for tenants with severe mental illness. They have office-based professional workers on site who are available, usually during office hours, to support tenants to maintain the tenancy and prevent homelessness. Secondly, independent tenancies with outreach support schemes. These are 'ordinary', private, local authority or housing association tenancies with regular visits from professional outreach workers to support tenants with severe mental illness in order to maintain the tenancy and prevent homelessness admissions.[5]

Support for carers
Focus on carers (see definition). Measures programmes aiming to alleviate workload for friends and relatives who voluntarily help people with a mental illness.

Systematic review (synonym: systematic overview)
A review of a clearly formulated question that uses systematic and explicit methods to identify, select and critically appraise relevant research, and to collect and analyse data from the studies that are included in the review. Statistical methods (meta-analysis) may or may not be used to analyse and summarise the results of the included studies. *See also* Cochrane Review.

User involvement
May include level of involvement (i.e. at executive board level, management level, clinical level (actual delivery of services); degree of influence on decision-making; level of funding; training and support for user groups.

LIST OF ABBREVIATIONS

ACT	Assertive community treatment
DARE	Database of abstracts of reviews of effectiveness
HMIC	Health management information consortium
CMHW	Community mental health worker
CMHT	Community mental health team
CPA	Care programme approach
CPN	Community Psychiatric Nurse
CRD	NHS Centre for Reviews and Dissemination
DOH	Department of Health
MHP	Mental health professional
NHS EED	NHS economic evaluation database
NSF	National Service Framework
PCG	Primary care group
OR	Odds ratio
RR	Relative risk

EXECUTIVE SUMMARY

BACKGROUND

The Government has recently developed a National Service Framework (NSF) for Mental Health. It covers the mental health needs of working age adults up to 65 and specifically addresses unacceptable variations in services across England. The Department of Health (DOH) commissioned the NHS Centre for Reviews and Dissemination (NHS CRD) to undertake a review of evidence on the cost-effectiveness of the mental health care services, based on the seven standards of the NSF for Mental Health.

PART 1. SCOPING REVIEW OF MENTAL HEALTH SERVICE DELIVERY INTERVENTIONS

The first part of this report (the scoping review of effectiveness) provides good information on systematic reviews of effectiveness and an insight into which areas have not been covered by recent (since 1994), good quality systematic reviews. It also links evidence from systematic reviews with the recommendations from the NSF.

Methodology

Search strategy

A comprehensive search strategy was developed. The Cochrane Library and the administrative version of DARE (Database of Abstracts of Reviews of Effectiveness) were searched. To ensure completeness, additional searches of PsycLIT (1999) and EMBASE (1994-2000) were undertaken. The Internet was also searched for relevant reviews.

Inclusion and exclusion criteria

Only Cochrane reviews or protocols, and systematic reviews published since 1994, which met strict quality criteria defined by NHS CRD, were included. Systematic reviews had to evaluate mental health promotion, or mental health service delivery/organisational interventions. Therapeutic interventions (e.g. pharmacological or psychological therapies compared with control) aimed at the individual were excluded. Participants in the reviews had to be adults aged 16 - 65 years with a mental health problem (e.g. depression, anxiety, neurosis, severe mental illness, eating disorders, deliberate self-harm or dual diagnosis). For mental health promotion interventions, subjects were the general adult population, some of whom may be at risk of developing mental health problems. Also included were reviews of carers of people with a mental health problem or dementia as they may be generalisable to other carers. Reviews of children, adolescents or people over 65 years of age (unless carers of people with a mental illness), people with mental disabilities such as Down's Syndrome (unless they also had a mental health problem), sex offenders and people with a personality disorder were excluded. Gaps in the evidence were identified through discussion with the Advisory Group, searching the Cochrane Controlled Trials Register for primary studies, consulting the topic lists from Cochrane Groups, and considering the examples of good practice in the NSF.

Data extraction and assessment of review quality

Initially titles and abstracts of the search results were independently screened for relevance by two reviewers. The full reports of all potentially relevant reviews were then independently assessed again by the two reviewers using the inclusion and exclusion criteria described previously. Data were then extracted from relevant reviews by one reviewer and checked by a second. To assess the variation in quality in reviews assumed to be of high quality, all completed reviews were assessed independently by two reviewers using the Oxman checklist. A score between one and seven was given for each review, with a score of one indicating major flaws, and a score of seven indicating minimal flaws.

RESULTS

Thirty-six completed systematic reviews and eight Cochrane protocols were included in this scoping review. Of the thirty-six reviews, nine were included in the NSF. This disparity may be due to the different search strategies used (the search strategy for the NSF was not described), the different objectives of the two documents and the fact that some reviews have been published since the NSF.

NSF standard 1: Mental health promotion
Mental health promotion was very difficult to define. Only one review, which specifically evaluated mental health promotion, was identified. As the outcome of interest in this area is often mental health and well-being, a range of environmental and social interventions as well as traditional health promotion interventions could be included in this section. Searching for all possible systematic reviews, however, was beyond the resources available for this scoping review. Areas not covered by systematic reviews include interventions to increase awareness and reduce the stigma of mental illness.

NSF Standards 2 and 3: Primary care and access to services
Seven systematic reviews and three protocols were identified. There are still gaps in the area of primary care, however, where systematic reviews have not been undertaken. Although the NSF recommends round the clock contact with the local services and the use of NHS direct, neither have been evaluated in systematic reviews. However, such interventions may be difficult to evaluate in systematic reviews

NSF standards 4 and 5: Effective services for people with severe mental illness
Twenty-one systematic reviews and five protocols were identified. The care programme approach is standard care in the UK and many of the recommendations for care of people with severe mental illnesses in the NSF are based on such an approach. Overall, the reviews concluded that ACT is an effective approach, and the care programme approach is less so. The NSF does, however, outline a national milestone which is to have assertive outreach in place for service users on enhanced CPA and at risk of losing contact with services. A further national milestone in the NSF is to increase the percentage of community mental health teams and the evidence from a Cochrane review suggests that this is an effective intervention.

One review evaluated crisis management, but no reviews have evaluated the effectiveness of the range of 24-hour services. However, such interventions will be difficult to evaluate (see Appendix 4). A number of good reviews exist on the effectiveness of specific services that provide 24-hour care. Further reviews of other specific services that provide 24-hour care may be considered after prudent prioritisation. Only one systematic review considered care within the hospital setting and concluded that short stay was more effective than long stay or standard care. No systematic reviews have been undertaken to evaluate interventions within the hospital setting such as home-like social environments.

NSF standard 6: Caring about carers
Four reviews were identified, but only one included carers of people with a mental illness. Although the needs of carers of people with dementia may be similar to those of people caring for someone with a mental illness, they were of lower quality than other reviews. Therefore, there is a need for further high quality systematic reviews to be undertaken in this area.

NSF standard 7: Preventing suicide
Three reviews evaluated primarily therapeutic interventions to reduce the rate of repeated self-harm and the risk of suicide. One of the national milestones of the NSF is for A&E departments to develop and implement protocols for those who present with self-harm. There are no systematic reviews specifically evaluating which protocols would be effective, but a Cochrane review is underway to evaluate primary and community health care professionals in hospital emergency departments and it may include relevant trials. No systematic reviews evaluating interventions to support local prison staff in preventing suicides among prisoners have been undertaken.

Conclusions

Thirty-six good quality systematic reviews have been undertaken and eight are being prepared in the areas of mental health promotion and mental health service delivery. Few of the systematic reviews, however, were able to conclude that an intervention was effective or not. This was due primarily to the poor quality, or limited amount of primary research. The only two interventions, which could be considered to be effective from the included primary research, were assertive outreach and community mental health teams. The care programme approach was not considered to be an effective intervention. For all of the other areas of mental health service delivery evaluated by the systematic reviews, interventions have been evaluated poorly, (or not at all) in the primary research.

There are still many areas of mental health service delivery interventions which have not been evaluated by systematic reviews including: services targeting more accurate diagnosis and assessment of common mental health problems; interventions within hospital settings, 24-hour staffed accommodation; more accurate assessment of risk of imminent violence (to self or others), and interventions for carers of people with a mental health problem. Only some included outcomes such as user's social networks, user and carer satisfaction, social relationships and quality of life. These outcomes should be incorporated into future systematic reviews and primary research. Undertaking systematic reviews in these areas will not only help to inform about what evidence is available, but can make recommendations for future primary research. It is recommended that Cochrane reviews should be undertaken where possible, but resources need to be available to keep them up-to-date.

PART 2. COST-EFFECTIVENESS OF MENTAL HEALTH SERVICE DELIVERY INTERVENTIONS

The second part of this report details the cost-effectiveness evidence from full economic evaluations of different modes of providing mental health services.

Methodology
Search strategy
Due to the limited time frame for the report, the NHS Economic Evaluation Database (NHS-EED) was the only source of economic evaluations. This database identifies studies from three databases: Current Contents-Clinical Medicine (1994 onwards), MEDLINE (1995 onwards) and CINAHL (1995 onwards). It also includes papers identified from handsearching the major biomedical journals and working papers from research centres specialising in health economics.

Inclusion and exclusion criteria
All relevant cost-effectiveness, cost-utility or cost-benefit studies. Methodological papers, discursive analysis of costs/benefits and partial evaluation studies were excluded. Inclusion and exclusion criteria for interventions and patient characteristics were the same as for part 1.

Data extraction
Two reviewers independently screened studies that met inclusion criteria, checking disagreements with a third reviewer.

Results
Twenty-seven studies met our inclusion criteria and were abstracted. These studies were grouped using the objectives of the NSF standards. Eighteen studies evaluated the cost-effectiveness of interventions in patients with a severe mental illness, eight evaluated interventions in primary care, and one evaluated interventions for carers of people with dementia. Twenty of the studies were randomised control studies (RCTs), four were non-RCTs and the rest were cohort, cross-sectional or before-after studies.

NSF standard one: Mental health promotion
No economic evaluations evaluating mental health promotion interventions were identified.

NSF standards two and three: Primary care and access to services
Eight studies evaluated the cost-effectiveness of interventions in the primary care setting; five studies evaluated the cost-effectiveness of community interventions for people with non-psychotic mental illnesses such as anxiety or depression. Four out of the five reported that

community care was more cost-effective than hospital or GP care. Two studies examined the cost-effectiveness of training GPs or providing guidelines for treating primary care somatising patients. Both were found to be cost-effective compared with standard care. One study estimated the cost-effectiveness of long-term specialised inpatient post-traumatic stress disorder (PTSD) units, relative to short-stay specialised PTSD units and to non-specialised general psychiatric units for the treatment of PTSD in Vietnam War veterans.

NSF standards 4 and 5: People with severe mental illness
Eighteen studies evaluated the cost-effectiveness of interventions for people with a severe mental illness. Seven were undertaken in the UK, eight in the USA, two in The Netherlands and one in Australia. Seven economic evaluations of community care compared with in-patient hospital care were identified. The types of interventions included: one study of outreach treatment; two studies of day care or day hospitals; two studies of types of accommodation; one study of a community training programme; and one study of short-term residential care. Overall, the majority reported that community interventions were more effective, or at least as effective as hospital care, and cheaper or no more expensive. The majority concluded that community care was a viable alternative to hospital care. Eleven economic evaluations also compared different types of community care.

One study compared a community support team with community psychiatric nurse teams, but found no difference in costs or effectiveness. Another study compared a modified therapeutic community with standard care, and found it to be more effective in improving psychological function but more expensive. A third study evaluated community care in three different regions in the USA and found community-based care to be more cost-effective than hospital-based care.

NSF standard 6: Caring for carers
One RCT looked at the cost-effectiveness of providing support to carers living with a relative with dementia but found no difference compared to community nursing.

NSF standard 7: Prevention of suicide
No economic evaluations evaluating interventions to prevent suicide were identified.

BACKGROUND

MENTAL HEALTH IN THE UK
Mental ill health is very common, and at any one time around one in six people of working age have a mental health problem, most often anxiety or depression. Furthermore, one person in 250 will have a psychotic illness such as schizophrenia or bipolar affective disorder (manic depression) and suicide is now the biggest cause of death among people under 35 years of age. Although suicide rates have started to decline, there are still around 4,000 deaths from suicide in England each year. One of the targets set out in 'Our Healthier Nation' is to reduce the death rate from suicide and undetermined injury by at least a fifth by 2010 - saving up to 4,000 lives in total.[6]

MODERNISING MENTAL HEALTH SERVICES IN THE UK
The Government's plans for improving mental health services for working age adults are set out in the paper, 'Modernising Mental Health Services, safe sound and supportive' published in December 1998.[7] An extra £700 million is to be made available over the next three years to improve the existing system, the quality and consistency of services and to develop closer working partnerships between the NHS and social services. Key measures include: more and better trained staff; early interventions; the provision of extra beds; better outreach facilities to ensure that health and local authorities deliver effective community treatment; 24 hour access to care and services (24 hour teams will stay in contact with patients in the community); good primary care; effective treatment and care processes; patients, service users and their carers to play an active role in the process of treatment and care; help to be provided where necessary to help people with mental health problems gain access to employment, education and housing services.

THE NATIONAL SERVICE FRAMEWORK FOR MENTAL HEALTH
The Government has more recently developed a National Service Framework (NSF) for Mental Health.[1] It covers the mental health needs of working age adults up to 65 and specifically addresses unacceptable variations in services across England.

The Framework:
- Sets national standards for both health and social care, and establishes performance indicators to measure the progress made by services, ensuring that they all meet basic criteria.
- Addresses the range of mental health service provision, from primary care, where the majority of mental health problems can be managed, through to specialist mental health services.
- Will help to ensure that people with mental health problems receive the service they need, regardless of who they are or where they live.

Local health and social care communities will agree local milestones with the NHS Executive regional offices and social care regions. An organisational framework for providing integrated services and for commissioning services is also included. The National Service Framework sets seven standards in five main areas:

Standard one	Mental health promotion
Standards two and three	Primary care and access to services
Standards four and five	Effective services for people with severe mental illness*
Standard six	Caring about carers
Standard seven	Preventing suicide

BACKGROUND AND RATIONALE FOR THE REVIEW
The Department of Health (DOH) commissioned the NHS Centre for Reviews and Dissemination (NHS CRD) to undertake a review of evidence on the cost-effectiveness of the mental health care services, based on the seven standards of the NSF for Mental Health.

---
* See glossary for the NSF working group definition of severe mental illness

After discussions between CRD and the DOH, however, it was decided that information on effectiveness needed to be ascertained before undertaking any review of cost-effectiveness. It was agreed, therefore, to undertake an initial scoping review of effectiveness, followed by a literature review of economic evaluations.

The first part of this report (the scoping review of effectiveness) provides:
- Good information on systematic reviews of effectiveness (which may be used by economists)
- Insight into which areas have not been covered by recent (since 1994), good quality systematic reviews
- Links between the evidence from reviews and the recommendations from the NSF

The second part of the report (a literature review of cost-effectiveness studies of mental health services) provides:
- Information on cost-effectiveness studies which have been undertaken in this area.

The scoping review will represent a starting point for further systematic reviews of effectiveness and may provide economic evaluations with best available effectiveness estimates. The literature review of economic evaluations of mental health service interventions will represent a starting point for work on modelling of needs, services, costs and outcomes.

REMIT OF THE REPORT
Both parts of this report concentrated on the types of care covered by the seven NSF standards. Evaluations of different types or locations of care and of care processes such as assessment and care management were the main focus. Evaluations of specific pharmaceutical or other therapeutic interventions were not included.

The DOH requested that the report focus on the following topics:
- Mental health promotion
- Diagnosis and treatment in primary care
- Assertive outreach
- Assessment, care management and care programmes
- Hospital inpatient and day patient care
- Community mental health teams
- 24 hour services
- Risk assessment
- Supported accommodation in the community
- Day care in the community, including the clubhouse model
- Employment opportunities
- Alternatives to secure accommodation
- Support for carers
- User involvement

PART 1. SCOPING REVIEW OF MENTAL HEALTH DELIVERY INTERVENTIONS

AIMS
To undertake a scoping review to identify good quality systematic reviews of mental health service delivery, and identify areas where no recent good quality systematic reviews have been undertaken.

OBJECTIVES
- To identify areas where good quality, up-to-date systematic reviews of the effectiveness of mental health services have been undertaken
- To identify areas where no good quality, up-to-date systematic reviews of the effectiveness of mental health services have been undertaken
- To compare the aims and recommendations from the NSF with the results and conclusions from systematic reviews
- To make recommendations for further systematic reviews

METHODS
Inclusion criteria
Only systematic reviews were included in this report. Such reviews are the most rigorous method of summarising a large body of literature in a critical and replicable way. They have a clearly formulated question that uses systematic and explicit methods to identify, select and critically appraise relevant research, and to collect and analyse data from the included studies. Statistical methods (meta-analysis) may or may not be used to analyse and summarise the results of the included studies.

All systematic reviews considered in this scoping review had to meet the following inclusion criteria for methodology of the review, interventions and participants:

1. Methodology of the reviews

Inclusion criteria
- Only good quality systematic reviews published since 1994 were included in this report. Cochrane reviews and systematic reviews that had met quality criteria set out by the NHS CRD in York, UK (see appendix 2) were included.

Exclusion criteria
- Reviews undertaken before 1994. Reviews published more than six years ago are likely to be out of date and may not reflect the current evidence.

2. Interventions evaluated in the reviews

Inclusion Criteria
- Mental health promotion
- Mental health service delivery/organisational interventions
- Different settings (e.g. inpatient vs outpatient) or methods of delivery (e.g. nurse vs doctor) for a therapeutic intervention

Exclusion Criteria
- Therapeutic interventions aimed at the individual (e.g. pharmacological or psychological therapies versus control or another therapeutic intervention)
- Educational or other interventions aimed at changing professional practice

3. Subjects included in the reviews

Inclusion Criteria
- Adults aged 16 - 65 years with a mental health problem (e.g. depression, anxiety, neurosis, severe mental illness, eating disorders, deliberate self-harm)
- For mental health promotion interventions, subjects were the general adult population, some of whom may be at risk developing mental health problems
- People with a dual diagnosis (e.g. drug/alcohol misuse and a mental illness)
- Carers of people with a mental health problem
- Carers of people with dementia (may be generalisable to other carers)

Exclusion Criteria
- Children, adolescents or people over 65 years of age (unless carers of people with a mental illness)
- People who abuse alcohol or drugs, unless they also have a mental health problem (i.e. dual diagnosis)
- People with mental disabilities such as Down's Syndrome
- Sex offenders
- People with a personality disorder

SEARCH STRATEGY
A comprehensive search strategy was developed by an experienced information specialist (KW) and is reported in detail in Appendix 1. Initially, The Cochrane Library and the administrative version of DARE (the Database of Abstracts of Reviews of Effectiveness) were searched. DARE provides coverage of the following databases: Current Contents (1994 to date); MEDLINE (1994 to date); CINAHL (1994 to date); AMED (1994 to 1998); ERIC (1995 to 1998); PsycLIT (1995 to 1998); BIOSIS (1996 to 1998). In addition, PsycLIT (1999), EMBASE (1994-2000) and the Internet were searched for relevant reviews.

APPLYING INCLUSION/EXCLUSION CRITERIA AND DATA EXTRACTION
Stage 1 - Applying inclusion and exclusion criteria
Initially titles and abstracts of the search results were independently screened for relevance by two reviewers (RJ and ZDB) who took an over-inclusive approach in order not to miss potentially relevant reports. Where there were disagreements about which reports appeared to be relevant, they were ordered as full paper copies. The full reports of all potentially relevant reviews were then independently assessed again by the two reviewers (RJ and ZDB) using the inclusion and exclusion criteria described previously. Any disagreements were resolved by an expert in the area (SG).

Stage 2 - Quality assessment
Cochrane reviews are considered to be the best available evidence, as they appear to have greater methodological rigour and are more frequently updated than systematic reviews or meta-analyses published in a paper format.[8] DARE reviews also have to meet a minimum set of quality criteria. However it may be that the quality varies within Cochrane reviews and also DARE reviews. To assess such variation in quality in reviews assumed to be of high quality, all reviews (not protocols) were assessed independently by two reviewers (RJ and ZDB) using the Oxman checklist for review articles.[9] A third reviewer (GtR) checked any reviews where there were disagreements.

Stage 3 - Data extraction
Data was extracted from relevant reviews into data extraction tables (see appendix 3) by one reviewer and checked by a second reviewer. If the review was included on DARE, information from the DARE record was extracted with additional information extracted as required. Any disagreements were resolved through discussion with a third reviewer (GtR).

Stage 4 - Reporting the results
Details of interventions, participants, and outcomes in the reviews were described both narratively and in tables in the results section of this report. Further information such as objectives, results and conclusions are reported in Appendix 3.

Stage 5 - Drawing conclusions and making recommendations
A list of areas that have been adequately covered by reviews was compiled, as well as a list of topic areas that have not been adequately reviewed (see boxes 2 and 3 at the end of the results section).

RESULTS
7557 references were retrieved and were independently scanned for relevance by two of the reviewers (RJ and ZDB). Of these, 135 were deemed to be relevant by either reviewer, but 39 of these were found to have already been excluded from DARE due to poor quality (i.e. not meeting the first of our inclusion criteria). Thus paper copies of 96 potentially relevant reviews were obtained. These 96 reviews were assessed independently by the two reviewers, using the inclusion and exclusion criteria described previously. Any disagreements were referred to an expert in the area (SG). The final number of included systematic reviews and systematic reviews in preparation was forty-four. Of these 11 were Cochrane reviews, three were journal publications of Cochrane reviews or protocols, 21 were published non-Cochrane reviews, one was an unpublished report and eight were in preparation (Cochrane protocols).

QUALITY OF INCLUDED REVIEWS
As mentioned previously, to be included in the review, all reviews had to be either Cochrane reviews, or meet the quality criteria for DARE. The methodological quality of the thirty-six reviews (14 Cochrane and 22 non-Cochrane) was assessed. One Cochrane protocol was published as a full review in a journal, and for the purposes of this report, it was considered to be a Cochrane review. Other Cochrane protocols were not assessed as they did not contain data, and therefore many of the Oxman criteria were not applicable (see box 1). Two reviewers independently assessed the methodological quality of the included reviews but were not blinded for the source of the reviews. Where there were differences (n=9), a third reviewer also independently assessed the quality and a consensus was reached. It was difficult to apply some of the criteria, especially to the non-Cochrane reviews. It is also recognised that there was some subjectivity in deciding on an overall score.

BOX 1
OXMAN QUALITY SCALE
1. Were the search methods to find evidence (original research) on the primary question(s) stated?
2. Was the search reasonably comprehensive?
3. Were the criteria used for deciding which studies to include in the overview reported?
4. Was bias in the selection of studies avoided?
5. Were the criteria used for assessing the validity of the included studies reported?
6. Was the validity of all studies assessed using appropriate criteria (either in selecting studies for inclusion or in analysing the studies cited)?
7. Were the methods used to combine the findings of the relevant studies (to reach a conclusion) reported?
8. Were the findings of the relevant studies combined appropriately relative to the primary question the overview addresses?
9. Were the conclusions made by the authors supported by the data and/or analysis reported in the overview?
10. How would you rate the scientific quality of this overview?

Extensive flaws		Major flaws		Minor flaws		Minimal flaws
1	2	3	4	5	6	7

Cochrane reviews scored consistently well on all of the Oxman criteria (see table 1). The fourteen Cochrane reviews scored between 5 and 7 points (minor or minimal flaws) and 10 of these scored the full 7 points. The 22 published reviews scored between 3 to 6 points (major to minor flaws) and none scored the full 7 points. There were two main areas in which most non-Cochrane reviews lacked methodological rigour and scored less well on the Oxman score. Firstly, the search strategy was often poorly defined, with few databases searched, and no attempt made to locate unpublished studies. Thus the possibility of publication bias is higher in these reviews. Publication bias is where the likelihood of publication is associated with the study's outcome (usually negative or inconclusive results). Because of this, systematic reviews that fail to include unpublished studies may overestimate the true effect of an intervention. In addition, some reviews only included English language studies, which means that important studies may have been missed. Secondly, some reviews did not contain an assessment of the quality of the included studies. Variation in quality can explain variation in the results of trials included in a systematic review. More rigorously designed (better 'quality') trials are more likely to yield results that are closer to the 'truth'. If this aspect of the study is not assessed, the conclusions of the review may be based on poor quality studies. If results are pooled the summary estimate may be biased and spuriously precise.

Table 1. Number of Cochrane and non-Cochrane reviews by quality score

Quality score		Cochrane reviews (n=14)	Published reviews (n=22)
High quality	7	10	0
	6	2	3
	5	2	8
	4	0	7
	3	0	4
	2	0	0
Low quality	1	0	0

All Cochrane reviews were published and/or updated since 1997 (see table 2). Although there were equal numbers of reviews published between 1997-1999 for both Cochrane and non-Cochrane reviews, five non-Cochrane reviews were published between 1995 and 1996. Thus these reviews will soon be out-of-date and new reviews may need to be written in these areas. In addition, each year, more and more published reviews will become out-of-date. For Cochrane reviews, the process of updating means that new evidence can be incorporated as it accrues. Once a topic area has been covered by a Cochrane review, therefore, other reviews to update the topic area probably do not need to be considered, unless they evaluate different outcomes or interventions.

Table 2. Number of Cochrane and non-Cochrane reviews by year published

Year published/ last updated	Cochrane reviews (n=14)	Published reviews (n=22)
2000	2	2
1999	6	8
1998	4	4
1997	2	3
1996	0	1
1995	0	4

1. NSF STANDARD ONE: MENTAL HEALTH PROMOTION

The NSF recommends that health and social services should:
1. promote mental health for all, working with individuals and communities
2. combat discrimination against individuals and groups with mental health problems, and promote their social inclusion

1. Promote mental health for all, working with individuals and communities

Mental health promotion is very difficult to define. The outcome of mental health and well-being is evaluated in a range of environmental and social interventions as well as traditional health promotion interventions. These environmental and social interventions may not refer specifically to mental health promotion although there may be an impact, either directly or indirectly, upon mental health Thus we agreed that searching for all possible systematic reviews was beyond the scope of the review. Instead we searched for reviews specifically evaluating mental health promotion interventions. Only one review was identified[10] and it defined mental health promotion as 'any activity undertaken with the goal of improving mental health or modifying its determinants or preventing mental illness or risk factors associated with it.' It reported that there was some evidence of the effectiveness of mass media interventions, general health promotion programmes, brief interventions at the time of critical illness, and 'listening visits'. Social support and problem solving or cognitive-behavioural training in the unemployed may improve mental health and employment outcomes. Many of these conclusions are drawn from the results of single studies, however, and should be interpreted with caution. Details of other systematic reviews that could fall under NSF standard one can be found in a document which contains a report on the national contract on mental health.[11] Important areas not covered by systematic reviews included interventions to increase awareness and reduce the stigma of mental illness.

2. Combat discrimination against individuals and groups with mental health problems, and promote their social inclusion

No systematic reviews were identified in this areas of reducing stigma and combating discrimination/social exclusion; increasing public awareness and understanding of mental health and mental illness; or developing healthy living centres.

Table 3. Details of systematic reviews relevant to NSF standard one*

Study details	Intervention	Primary outcomes	Results	Quality score[#]	Comments
Tilford 1997[10]	Mental health promotion for the general population and high risk groups	Promotion of positive mental health, prevention of specified mental disorders and outcomes	Many different interventions and population groups. See text for more details of results	5	*Comments on review:* Only English language studies published between 1980 and 1995 included. *Comments on primary studies:* Most results based on single studies

- For Cochrane reviews, year review was last updated

[#] Adapted from Oxman et al[9]: 1= extensive flaws, 7= minimal flaws in the review

Further details of this review are provided in Appendix 3

2. NSF STANDARDS TWO AND THREE: PRIMARY CARE AND ACCESS TO SERVICES

The NSF recommends that any service user who contacts their primary health care team with a common mental health problem should:
1. Have their mental health needs identified and assessed
2. Be offered effective treatments, including referral to specialist services for further assessment treatment and care if they require it

Any individual with a common mental health problem should:
3. Be able to make contact round the clock with the local services
4. Be able to use NHS direct

In addition, NSF milestones and recommendations include:
5. A&E departments should have liaison arrangements
6. Primary Care Groups (PCGs) will need to develop the resources to work with diverse groups in the population
7. PCGs should agree and implement assessment and management protocols across the primary care group for people with depression, postnatal depression, eating disorders, anxiety disorders, and for people with schizophrenia

1. Identification and assessment of mental health needs

One systematic review evaluated interventions to improve the recognition and/or management of mental disorders by health care professionals in the primary care setting.[12] Results suggested that such interventions may improve the diagnosis, treatment and clinical outcomes of depression and other mental disorders in primary care. The other review (both a published review,[13] and a Cochrane protocol[14]) evaluated interventions aimed at improving primary prevention in general, not just related to mental health. Although only one relevant trial was included in the published review, and few details were provided, any future trials in this area will be included in the Cochrane review. There were no systematic reviews of diagnosis and assessment of mental illness in primary care (i.e. diagnostic tools).

2. Referral to specialist services for further assessment treatment and care

One systematic review (both a published review,[15] and also a Cochrane protocol[16]) found some support for the hypothesis that on-site mental health workers (MHWs) produce short term reductions in psychotropic prescribing and mental health referrals. However, the effects were inconsistent and may not persist over time. Two Cochrane reviews are underway to evaluate interventions to provide care for new attenders at the hospital emergency department[17] and interventions to change or improve referrals from primary care physicians to secondary care.[18] Both reviews will focus on health care in general, not specifically mental health services. However, studies of people with a mental illness will be included if they are relevant to the reviews.

3. 'Round the clock' contact with the local services

No systematic reviews evaluating the effectiveness of round the clock contact were identified.

4. Helplines including NHS Direct

No systematic reviews evaluating the effectiveness of telephone helplines were identified.

5. Liaison within A&E

No systematic reviews have evaluated the effectiveness of liaison within A&E, but a review is underway to evaluate interventions in which primary or community care professionals provide care for new attenders at the hospital emergency department.[17] The focus is not on people with a mental health problem, but will include relevant studies if they meet the inclusion criteria.

6. Developing the resources to work with diverse groups in the population

No systematic reviews to evaluate resources to work with diverse groups in the population were identified.

7. Assessment and management protocols for depression, postnatal depression, eating disorders, anxiety disorders, and for people with schizophrenia.

One systematic review evaluated professional and/or social support interventions for postpartum depression.[19] The review concluded that there is some indication that professional and/or social support (counselling from health care professionals) may help in the treatment of postpartum depression. It should be noted, however, that the review only contained two small trials (n=111). No systematic reviews to date have evaluated health service delivery interventions for anorexia nervosa and other eating disorders. A Cochrane review is underway, however, to evaluate anorexia nervosa specialist clinics versus non-specialist clinics.[20]

One review evaluated interventions to help patients follow prescriptions for medications.[21] This was a review covering all patients not just those with a mental illness. The author concluded that current methods of improving adherence for chronic health problems are mostly complex and not very effective.

General guideline literature on the management of depression of primary care was not evaluated in this review. An *Effective Health Care* Bulletin on the treatment of depression in primary care, however, was published in 1993,[22] and is presently being updated.

Areas of diagnosis and management not covered by systematic reviews include:
- increasing knowledge about self help and self-help groups
- more generic approaches to managing prescribing in primary care
- detection vs. disclosure on outcome of depression in general practice
- liaison psychiatry/psychiatrists/other mental health professionals in primary care settings
- case management of depression by clinical pharmacists in a primary care setting
- one stop shop clinics

Table 4. Details of systematic reviews relevant to NSF standards two and three*

	Study details	Intervention	Primary outcomes	Results	Quality score[#]	Comments
Identification and assessment of mental health needs	Hulscher 1999[13,14]	Improving primary prevention	Any objective measure of professional performance or patient health outcomes	Only one study was relevant and few details were provided	6	*Comments on review*: Also a Cochrane protocol so more information may become available in the future from relevant primary studies
	Kroenke 2000[12]	Recognition and/or management of mental disorders	Provider knowledge, attitudes or skill, process of care, and clinical outcomes	Interventions aimed at recognition/management: ↑[b] diagnosis ↔[b] clinical improvement in psychiatric symptoms or functional status	5	*Comments on review*: No formal quality assessment of included studies. *Comments on primary studies*: 27 RCTs, and 21 non-RCTs (n=27,284) but not all relevant. Heterogeneity in interventions and outcomes.
Referral to specialist services for further assessment treatment and care	Abi-Aad 2000[17]	Primary or community care professionals in A&E department	Diagnostic interventions, treatments, referrals to specialist care, hospital admission	N/A	N/A	*Comments on review*: Cochrane protocol (expected end 2001)
	Bower 2000*[15,16]	On-site mental health workers (MHW)	Detection rates and diagnostic accuracy, off-site mental health referral behaviour, PCP prescribing behaviour	Compared with standard care, MHW: ↓[b] psychotropic prescribing and mental health referral ↓[b] consultation rates Short term effects/inconsistent results	7	*Comments on review*: Methodologically sound *Comments on primary studies*: 38 controlled and uncontrolled studies (n=3880), but insufficient studies available to provide reliable estimates. Inadequate and inconsistent reporting of data
	Grimshaw 1999[18]	Referral from primary to secondary care	Objective measures of provider performance (e.g. referral rates)	N/A	N/A	*Comments on review*: Cochrane protocol (was expected end 2000)
Setting of care, assessment and management protocols	Boyle 1999[20]	Setting of care for anorexia nervosa	Morgan Russell scale which considers all facto's in addition to Body Mass Index alone	N/A	N/A	*Comments on review*: Cochrane protocol (was expected mid-2000)
	Schulberg 1998[23]	Setting of care for depression	Effectiveness in treating depression	When transferred from psychiatric to primary care settings, antidepressants: ↓[b] depression	4	*Comments on review*: Only included studies published between 1992 and 1998. No quality assessment of included studies. *Comments on primary studies*: Number of studies not stated.
	Ray 1997*[19]	Professional and/or social support for women with post-natal depression	Duration and resolution of the depression; social functioning	Compared with standard care, professional and/or social support: ↓[a] depression	7	*Comments on review*: Methodologically sound *Comments on primary studies*: Only two small RCTs (n=137) were relevant for inclusion
	Haynes 1999*[21]	Interventions to affect adherence with prescribed, self-administered medications	Medication adherence and treatment outcome	Simple and complex interventions: ↑[b] adherence but not greatly ↔[b] clinical outcomes	5	*Comments on review*: No clear quality assessment of included studies *Comments on primary studies*: Only 5 studies (n=not stated) related to schizophrenia and other mental illnesses

* For Cochrane reviews, year review was last updated
[#] Adapted from Oxman et al [9]. 1= extensive flaws, 7= minimal flaws in the review; ↓ decrease in outcome as compared with standard care/comparison intervention; ↑ increase in outcome as compared with standard care/comparison intervention
↔ no difference in outcome between groups, or insufficient data to detect a difference
[a] results from pooled meta-analysis. Results significant at p<0.05; [b] results from narrative synthesis of results. Meta-analysis not performed due to clinical or statistical heterogeneity
Further details of these reviews are provided in Appendix 3

3. NSF STANDARDS FOUR AND FIVE: EFFECTIVE SERVICES FOR PEOPLE WITH SEVERE MENTAL ILLNESS

The NSF for mental health recommends that all mental health service users on the care programme approach (CPA) should:
1. Receive care which optimises engagement, anticipates or prevents a crisis and reduces risk
2. Have a copy of a written care plan
3. Be able to access services 24 hours a day, 365 days a year

Those service users who are assessed as having a period of care away from home should have:
4. Timely access to an appropriate hospital bed which is in the least restrictive environment and as close to home as possible
5. A copy of a written care plan agreed on discharge

In addition, the NSF suggest that:
6. Specific measures may be needed to engage people with co-morbidity

Milestones include:
7. Assessment and access to services for those coming into contact with the criminal justice system
8. Access to education, training, occupational and social care support, including supported accommodation
9. The use of high and medium secure beds, availability of intensive care beds, crisis and refuge places, 24 hour staffed places, hostel places and other supported residential places

Twenty-one systematic reviews (one an unpublished HTA monograph) have been undertaken to assess the effectiveness of health service delivery interventions for people with severe mental illnesses (see table 5). Five more Cochrane reviews are underway. Several of these evaluated the same interventions, such as case management and assertive outreach. Thus they may have included similar trials. More details including results and conclusions are to be found in Appendix 3.

1. Receiving care which optimises engagement, anticipates or prevents a crisis and reduces risk

Optimising engagement - community mental health teams, and community mental health nurses

One of the national milestones in the NSF is to increase the percentage of community mental health teams. One Cochrane review assessed the effectiveness of CMHTs[24] and concluded that CMHT management is not inferior to non-team standard care in any important respect and is superior in promoting greater acceptance of treatment. The authors concluded the findings give some general support to the case for establishing and maintaining CMHTs as a corner stone of mental health policy. However, data relating to clinical outcomes and pattern of hospital care is unsatisfactory. CMHTs, however, have no apparent disadvantages and may decrease hospitalisation. A further systematic review reported that people receiving care from community mental health nurses (CMHN) were less depressed and reported better general health than people receiving standard care.[25]

Optimising engagement - care programme approach

Four systematic reviews (three non-Cochrane and one Cochrane reviews) evaluated case management or care management for people with a severe mental illness.[2,26-28] Definitions for these interventions varied between studies. For example, the Cochrane review included any studies that described the intervention as 'case management' in the trial report and the UK terms 'care management' and 'care programme approach' were treated as synonyms for case management.[2] One of the non-Cochrane reviews described it as either 'brokerage case management (focusing on the organisation and co-ordination of services on behalf of the client) or clinical case management (assertive community treatment, the psychosocial rehabilitation model and the strengths model).[26] Another evaluated a number of different case management approaches defined as standard case management (broker and clinical case management), assertive community treatment, intensive case management, strengths case management and rehabilitation case management.[27] The last review evaluated a combination of one or more of three models of 'innovative care': multidisciplinary teams, home care and case management. Comparison was conventional care.[28] The most common outcomes were related to use of service (e.g. hospital admissions), but one did evaluate quality of care.[28]

One Cochrane review comparing case management (care programme approach) with standard care found although it increased contact with services, it had no other advantages and increased hospital use.[2] In terms of costs, it was expensive from a health care perspective, but cost-effective from a societal perspective. The authors concluded that case management is an intervention of questionable value, to the extent that it is doubtful whether it should be offered by community psychiatric services. At the present time CPA is standard care in the UK.

Optimising engagement - assertive community treatment
A further national milestone outlined in the NSF is to have assertive outreach in place for service users on enhanced CPA and at risk of losing contact with services. Two non-Cochrane reviews and one Cochrane review evaluated assertive community treatment (ACT) and/or assertive case management.[29-31] Two described their definition of the intervention as being based on the Madison, Treatment in Community Living, Assertive Community Treatment or Stein and Test models.[29,30] The third used a number of items to decide whether the programmes used in the studies were of high fidelity.[31] Programmes were coded as being of 'high fidelity' if, in addition to following a shared-caseload model and providing the majority of services in the community, they explicitly met at least four of the following five criteria: 1) staff:client ratio of 1:12 or better; 2) a psychiatrist on staff; 3) at least one nurse on staff; 4) at least some coverage outside of normal working hours; 5) at least two team meetings every week. The results of the systematic reviews indicated that the most effective community-based service in reducing hospital use appears to be assertive community treatment (ACT).[29-31] ACT was also reported to have moderate effects in improving symptomatology and quality of life,[32] increasing the chances of employment,[30] housing stability[27,30] and satisfaction.[31] Unlike case management, ACT emphasises team working and team responsibility and has been based on American models. Since these services have a number of components, interventions incorporating a larger number of elements have been defined as 'high fidelity' programmes. These have been shown to be more effective than lower fidelity services.[31] One review also reported that the whole ACT model rather than selective elements appears to be more effective.[30] It should be noted that most of the research in this area was undertaken in the USA, and may not be generalisable to the UK setting. At the present time, no systematic reviews are evaluating consumer led ACT vs. standard ACT.

One other systematic review in preparation evaluated all types of home treatment for people with severe mental illness. However, the only outcome assessed was hospital days.[33] The review concluded that it was difficult to reach conclusions on either effectiveness or cost-effectiveness.

Areas of community care package/setting of care not fully covered by systematic reviews include:
- Acute day hospital + crisis respite programme
- Community mental health centres
- Guardianship networks
- Subsidised housing
- Telephone follow up
- Community interventions such as: care post-discharge and visits of different frequencies

Optimising care- crisis interventions
One Cochrane review evaluated crisis interventions for people with severe mental illness. These were defined as any type of crisis-orientated treatment of an acute psychiatric episode by staff with a specific remit to deal with such situations, in and beyond 'office hours'. The

comparison was standard care, which was defined as the normal care given to those suffering from acute psychiatric episodes in the area concerned. Studies comparing different models of 'crisis intervention', mobile and non-mobile units, were also utilised in a second comparison within the review.[34] The authors concluded that home care crisis treatment, coupled with an ongoing home care package, is a viable and acceptable way of treating people with serious mental illnesses. More clinically effective packages may have already eclipsed crisis intervention but if crisis intervention policy is to be practised or implemented it would be hard to justify this outside of a simple well-designed trial. Issues such as staff satisfaction and burnout would also be important. They also recommended that policy makers should be wary of using resources purely for short-term crisis intervention packages until further information is available. Further systematic reviews of other crisis interventions may be warranted.

2. Patient holding a copy of a written plan

One Cochrane review examined the effectiveness of patients with psychotic illnesses holding clinical information, but no studies met the inclusion criteria (see table 3).[35] One study was identified but it was not randomised, and two others RCTs are ongoing. The authors concluded that there is a gap in the evidence regarding patient-held, personalised, accessible clinical information for people with psychotic illnesses. It cannot be assumed that patient-held information is beneficial or cost-effective without evidence from well-planned, conducted and reported randomised trials.

3. 24-hour care

Evaluating the effectiveness of 24-hour care is difficult because of the wide range of interventions that include such cover. Services differ in the way care is provided outside of office hours, from on call staff providing immediate response to an automated 24-hour telephone helpline asking callers to call back during office hours. No systematic reviews evaluating 24-hour care have been undertaken, but a paper on the feasibility of such reviews has been prepared (see Appendix 4).

4. Time spent in hospital and hospital care

The NSF suggested that short a stay in hospital might improve care and outcomes especially with good quality care and rapid follow up. One Cochrane review evaluated the effect of planned short stay admission policies versus a long or standard stay for people with serious mental illnesses (see table 3).[36] The authors concluded that planned short stays seemed to be as successful, or more so than standard care: patients experienced no more admissions and no more losses to follow up and were more likely to be discharged on time. No systematic reviews have been undertaken which evaluate interventions within the hospital setting (e.g. homelike social environment). Furthermore no systematic reviews have been undertaken of intensive 24-hour staffed residential and nursing homes.

Systematic reviews are currently being conducted to evaluate the effectiveness of day centres, day hospitals and supported housing schemes.[17,37]

One of the aims of the NSF is that hospital beds are in the least restrictive environment consistent with the need to protect them and the public. One systematic review hypothesised that it was possible, in acute clinical settings, to predict with reasonable accuracy which patients are most likely to become aggressive or violent in the near future.[38] The quality of the included data was not high, and there was no clear consensus on items useful for prediction of violence.

Areas under this heading not covered by systematic reviews include:
- therapies and interventions WITHIN residential units or hospital wards (e.g. homelike social environment)
- scheduled intermittent or long-term hospitalisation
- rapid discharge programme
- intensive guideline implementation intervention
- quality of acute care
- home care with 24 hour staffing
- discharge planning and communication with community health services

5. Copy of a written care plan agreed on discharge
See section 2.

6. Dual Diagnosis
The NSF suggests that mental health and drugs and alcohol services should meet the needs of people with a dual diagnosis (see table 3). Two reviews evaluated the effectiveness of interventions for substance abusers with severe mental illnesses.[39,40] Both reviews found that studies in these areas were of poor methodology. The Cochrane review concluded that there was not enough evidence that extra resources, required to deliver substance misuse treatment integrated with mental health care for people with severe mental health problems, will lead to benefit.[39]

7. Assessment and access to services for those coming into contact with the criminal justice system
Two systematic reviews evaluated interventions within the criminal justice system for people with mental illnesses. One systematic review evaluated interventions/regimes in services for women assessed as needing psychiatric care in conditions of security.[41] Only one small cohort study was identified examining the effectiveness of psychiatric care. This study found a poorer outcome amongst women admitted from psychiatric hospital compared with women admitted from courts. The other systematic review evaluated studies of secure, and non-secure democratic therapeutic communities, for people with personality disorders, and mentally disordered offenders.[42] Although the authors searched for all studies relating to therapeutic communities, the majority was for people with personality disorders, rather than other severe mental illnesses. The review reported that, although there is evidence that therapeutic communities produce changes in people's mental health and functioning, further research is needed. It is worth noting that a previous CRD report is a scoping review of literature on the health and care of mentally disordered offenders.[43]

8. Access to education, training, occupational and social care support, including supported accommodation
Many of these interventions fall outside the remit of this review. Two reviews, however, evaluated vocational rehabilitation programmes such as supported employment.[44,45] Both reviews found that such interventions appear to be promising approaches for people with severe mental illness, but more studies are needed, with close attention to programme implementation and long-term follow-up. Although the conclusions appeared to follow on from the results, both reviews had methodological flaws. A Cochrane review of vocational rehabilitation is also, however, is being prepared using more rigorous methodology.[46]

One review evaluated life skills programmes.[47] The authors concluded that if life skills training is to continue as part of rehabilitation programmes, a large, well designed, conducted and reported pragmatic randomised trial is needed. There may even be an argument for stating that maintenance of current practice, outside of a randomised trial, is unethical.

Further Cochrane reviews are underway to evaluate supported housing schemes or outreach support schemes[5], day care centres[37] and day hospitals.[48]

9. The use of high and medium secure beds, availability of intensive care beds, crisis and refuge places, 24 hour staffed places, hostel places and other supported residential places
No systematic reviews have been undertaken to evaluate interventions in this area. Areas where reviews may be considered include:
- use of high and medium secure beds
- crisis and refuge places (although there is a review of crisis intervention; see point 1)
- 24 hour staffed places (see also point 4)
- hostel places and other supported residential places (although interventions to evaluate supported housing are being evaluated, see point 8)

Table 5. Details of systematic reviews relevant to NSF standards four and five*

	Study details	Intervention	Primary outcomes	Results	Quality score[#]	Comments
Care which optimises engagement, anticipates or prevents a crisis and reduces risk	Brooker 1996[25]	Community mental health nurses	Depression, anxiety, fear, general health, hopelessness, social adjustment and process measures	Compared to standard care, CMHN: ↓[b] depression ↑[b] self-esteem and general health ↑[b] satisfaction	5	*Comments on review*: Focused on methodological quality of studies. Little emphasis given to the actual effectiveness of CMHN interventions. Also limited information about included studies *Comments on primary studies*: 10 small poor quality RCTs and quasi-RCTs (n=670)
	Wadhwa 1999[28]	Multidisciplinary teams, home care and case management	Quality of care	Compared to standard care, multidisciplinary outreach strategies: ↓[b] hospitalisation	5	*Comments on review*: Only English language studies included *Comments on primary studies*: 14 RCTs (n=2,161), but heterogeneous interventions
	Tyrer 1999*[24]	Community mental health teams (CMHTs)	Death, violence, acceptability of management as measured by loss to follow up, and general improvement.	Compared to standard care, CMHTs: ↓[a] suicide rates ↑[a] satisfaction ↓[a] leaving study early (drop-outs) ↔[b] hospitalisation/ clinical outcomes	6	*Comments on review*: Methodologically sound *Comments on primary studies*: 5 RCTs (n=869). Poorly presented data on hospitalisation and clinical outcomes
Assertive Community Treatment (ACT) and case/care management)	Holloway 1995[26]	ACT+ case management, brokerage case management and clinical	Hospital days and admissions, costs, use of community care services, satisfaction with services, quality of life, symptoms, social functioning	Compared with standard case management, case management + ACT: ↓[b] length and rate of hospitalisation ↑[b] compliance rates ↔[b] symptomatology	4	*Comments on review*: Strength of evidence not based on the study quality. Only one database searched. *Comments on primary studies*: 23 studies (n=3,803). Wide range of definitions, little attempt to tease out key components and unstandardised outcome measures
	Latimer 1999[31]	ACT, both high and low fidelity	Time spent in hospital, costs, independent housing	Compare with control, ACT: ↓[b] independent housing ↓[b] costs for high service users ↔ Supervised housing costs Compared with low fidelity ACT, high fidelity ACT: ↓[b] hospital use	3	*Comments on review*: Limited number of studies reviewed. Literature search not well-defined. Quality of trials not assessed apart from fidelity to ACT model. Primarily assessing economic issues *Comments on primary studies*: 19 RCTs and 15 non-RCTs (n=4,791)
	Marshall 1998*[30]	ACT and assertive case management	Remaining in contact with psychiatric services, extent of psychiatric hospital admissions, clinical and social outcome and costs	Compared with standard care, ACT: ↓[a] hospital use ↑[a] independent accommodation, ↑[a] employment ↑[a] satisfaction in ACT group ↔[a] mental state and social functioning ↓[b] costs for high service users ↔[b] all costs	7	*Comments on review*: Methodologically sound *Comments on primary studies*: 20 RCTs (n=3502). Insufficient data to compare ACT with case management and difficult to draw a clear distinction between them. Mostly USA studies.
	Mueser 1998[27]	ACT compared with standard case management and other models of case management	Time in hospital, symptoms, social adjustment, housing stability, substance abuse, medication compliance, quality of life, vocational functioning, patient/relative satisfaction	Compared with standard care, ACT: ↓[b] length of hospital stay ↑[b] housing stability (in high service users) ↓[b] symptomatology (moderate) ↑[b] quality of life	5	*Comments on review*: Authors do not state which databases they searched, nor search terms or dates. No quality assessment of included studies. *Comments on primary studies*: Included 75 studies of which 32 were RCTs (n= not stated). Mostly USA studies.

Study details	Intervention	Primary outcomes	Results	Quality score[#]	Comments
Scott 1995[29]	ACT (as described by Stein and Test)	Use of inpatient hospitalisation and community mental health services, costs and clinical and social outcome	Compared with standard case management, case management + ACT: ↓[b] rate and duration of hospitalisation ↑[b] use of community mental health services	4	*Comments on review:* Only two databases searched. No quality assessment of included studies. *Comments on primary studies:* 7 reviews and 12 RCTs (n=1,789). Difficult to discern the border between ACT and intensive case management
Marshall 1997*[2]	Case management (UK terms 'care management' and 'care programme approach')	Numbers remaining in contact with the psychiatric services, extent of psychiatric hospital admissions, clinical and social outcomes, and costs	Compared with standard care, case management/CPA: ↑[a] hospital admissions (double) ↑[b] contact with services (small effect) ↑[b] compliance (one study) ↔[a] mental state, social functioning, quality of life ↔[b] Costs may be higher but insufficient evidence	7	*Comments on review:* Methodologically sound *Comments on primary studies:* 11 RCTs (n=1,642). Insufficient data available on costs
Crisis interventions					
Joy 2000*[34]	Crisis interventions	Hospitalisation, patient, carer and staff satisfaction with treatment, clinical outcomes (e.g. death/suicide, improvement), social functioning and economic costs	Compared with standard care, crisis intervention: ↓[a] repeat admissions (small decrease) ↓[a] loss to follow up at 6 months ↓[a] family burden ↑[b] satisfaction for patients & family ↔[a] loss to follow-up, death or mental state ↑[b] All studies found it to be more cost-effective, but data unusable	7	*Comments on review:* Methodologically sound *Comments on primary studies:* Five RCTs (n=764). Studies of 'pure' crisis interventions not available. Crisis interventions usually coupled with ongoing package of care. 24-hour care ranged from telephone answering machine to staff on call.
Other home based care					
Burns 2000[33] Ongoing	Home based care	Hospital stay	Difficult to reach conclusions on either effectiveness or cost-effectiveness	5	*Comments on review:* HTA monograph in press *Comments on primary studies:* 56 RCTs and 35 non-RCTs (n=not stated). Poorly presented data, highly heterogeneous interventions.
Prompts					
Reda 2000[49]	Prompts to encouraging appointment attendance	Service utilisation and compliance	N/A	N/A	*Comments on review:* Cochrane protocol (expected mid-2001)
Patient holding a copy of a written plan					
Henderson 1999*[35]	Patient-held information	Hospital admission, death from causes other than suicide, violence to self or others	No included studies	7	*Comments on review:* Methodologically sound *Comments on primary studies:* Two important RCTs are ongoing, and results will be included in future updates
Time spent in hospital and hospital care					
Johnstone 1999[36,50]	Planned short stay/brief admission to hospital	Relapse, readmission, death, violent incidents, loss to follow up, discharge, mental state, social functioning, patient satisfaction, family burden	Compared with long stays, short stays: ↔[a] readmissions ↔[a] losses to follow-up ↑[a] successful discharge on time	7	*Comments on review:* Methodologically sound. Cochrane and published review. Results taken from published review, as more up to date *Comments on primary studies:* 4 RCTs (n=628) published in the 1970's, most undertaken in the USA
Wing 1998[38]	Prediction of imminent violence	Accuracy in the prediction assessment of violence	↔[b] no clear consensus on items that would be clinically useful for short-term prediction	5	*Comments on review:* Primarily a guideline document. *Comments on primary studies:* 16 poor quality non controlled studies (n=not stated). Heterogeneity in settings, patients and predictive instruments

	Study details	Intervention	Primary outcomes	Results	Quality score[#]	Comments
Time spent within the criminal justice system	Lees 1999[42]	Therapeutic communities	Mental health and functioning, recidivism, re-admission and relapse	Compared with control, therapeutic communities: ↑[a] recidivism, re-admission and relapse	5	*Comments on review:* No clear validity assessment and difficult to interpret meta-analysis *Comments on primary studies:* 52 studies (n= not stated), mainly of people with personality disorders
	Lart 1999[41]	Interventions/regimes for women assessed as needing subsequent psychiatric care in conditions of security.	Progress, based on psychiatric condition, behaviour, work record, further court appearances and re-admissions.	Only one small study identified	6	*Comments on review:* Partial validity assessment *Comments on primary studies:* Only one small cohort study (n=33) identified
Access to education, training, occupational and social care support. *Vocational rehabilitation*	Bond 1997[44]	Vocational programmes offering supported employment	Employment rate	Compare with control, vocational employment ↑[b] employment rates ↔[b] no evidence of increased hospitalisation	4	*Comments on review:* Search terms not described. No quality assessment of included studies. *Comments on primary studies:* 21 studies (n=1873). Only one RCT found. Heterogeneity in models and outcomes. Unclear definitions of specific components
	Crowther 1999[46]	Vocational rehabilitation	Number of people in competitive employment at end of the study	N/A	N/A	*Comments on review:* Cochrane protocol (expected mid-2000)
	Lehman 1995[45]	Vocational rehabilitation	Vocational functioning	Compared with control, vocational rehabilitation: ↑[b] employment rates (whilst on programme) ↓[b] hospital admissions	3	*Comments on review:* Only two databases searched. No assessment of study quality. *Comments on primary studies:* 24 controlled trials (n=2,715). Number of trials for each model was small.
Day hospitals or day care	Almaraz-Serrano 1997[48]	Day hospital care or day time attendance at a facility	Contact with services, extent of hospital care received, clinical and social outcomes, costs of care	N/A	N/A	*Comments on review:* Cochrane protocol (expected mid-2000)
	Catty 1999[37]	Day centre care	Mortality, leaving study early, clinical response, violent or criminal behaviour, service use, costs, quality of life / satisfaction	N/A	N/A	*Comments on review:* Cochrane protocol (expected mid-2000)
Supported housing	Hayes 1997[5]	Supported housing schemes or outreach support schemes	Service utilisation, medical/mental state changes, professional support workers' and user satisfaction, social functioning, quality of life, economic outcomes	N/A	N/A	*Comments on review:* Cochrane protocol (expected mid-2000)
Life skills	Nicol 1998*[47]	Life skills programmes	Self-care functioning at personal and domestic level (life skills)	Compare with control, life skills programmes: ↔[b] life skills. Data were sparse and no clear effects	7	*Comments on review:* Methodologically sound *Comments on primary studies:* Only two RCTs (n=38) identified

	Study details	Intervention	Primary outcomes	Results	Quality score[#]	Comments
Dual Diagnosis	Drake 1998[40]	Integrated treatments that combined mental health and substance abuse treatments	Engagement in treatment, substance use behaviours and outcomes, hospital utilisation and symptoms of mental illness	Overall, compared to standard care dual diagnosis programmes: ↔[b] Inconsistent findings Some evidence that long-term comprehensive integrated dual-disorder programmes: →[b] substance abuse →[b] readmission rates →[b] hospital use ↑[b] clinical outcomes	5	*Comments on review*: No quality assessment of included studies. *Comments on primary studies*: 36 controlled and uncontrolled studies (n=not stated). Poor methodology of included studies. Comprehensive integrated dual disorder programmes consist of a large number of elements (motivational interviewing, assertive outreach, intensive case management, individual counselling, family interventions).
	Ley 1999*[39]	Programmes of substance misuse treatment within standard psychiatric care	Numbers lost to treatment, symptoms of severe mental illness, substance use, hospitalisation	↔[b] No clear evidence due to poor methodology ↔[b] No evidence that one programme is superior to another	7	*Comments on review*: Methodologically sound *Comments on primary studies*: 6 RCTs (n= 659) Lack of evidence may also be due to high drop out rates

* For Cochrane reviews, year review was last updated
# Adapted from Oxman et al 9. 1= extensive flaws, 7= minimal flaws in the review
→ decrease in outcome as compared with standard care/comparison intervention.
↑ increase in outcome as compared with standard care/comparison intervention
↔ no difference in outcome between groups, or insufficient data to detect a difference
[a] Results significant at p<0.05
[a] results from pooled meta-analysis.
[b] results from narrative synthesis of results. Meta-analysis not performed due to clinical or statistical heterogeneity

Further details of these reviews are provided in Appendix 3

4. NSF STANDARD SIX: CARING ABOUT CARERS

> All individuals who provide regular and substantial care for a person on CPA should:
> 1. Have an assessment of their caring, physical and mental health needs, repeated on at least an annual basis
> 2. Have their own written care plan which is given to them and implemented in discussion with them

Four reviews were included in this section (see table 6). Reviews of carers of people with dementia were included, as they may be generalisable to carers of people with mental illness.

1. Have an assessment of their caring, physical and mental health needs, repeated on at least an annual basis

Family interventions

One systematic review evaluated family interventions.[51] These ranged from one educational session to intensive family treatment. The review concluded that interventions such as information giving, discussion, sharing and coping strategies with at least ten sessions can have considerable effects on relatives' burden, relatives' psychological distress, the relationship between the patient and the relative, and family functioning. Systematic reviews evaluating other interventions aimed at carers of people with mental health are required. Also systematic reviews of the effectiveness of written care plans and needs assessment, checklists for GPs and primary care teams to help carers may be warranted.

Respite care

Two systematic reviews evaluated the effectiveness of respite care for carers of people with dementia.[52, 53] One review categorised respite care under four main headings: 'inpatient' residential respite care, out of home 'day care, out of home 'overnight' care and 'in home' respite (which usually involved scheduled visits from a nurse/care assistant).[53] Outcomes assessed included carer's well-being, burden of care, carer's quality of life and carer's physical health. Both reported that the majority of the studies in this area were methodologically poor and that there was little evidence that respite care for a patient with dementia significantly affects caregiver burden or delays institutionalisation of the patient. In addition, one reported that the carer's attitude toward the patient was worse after respite.[52]

Other interventions

The Cochrane review evaluated many other interventions for carers such as individualised service assessment and planning versus conventional care or no support; technology-based networking versus conventional care or no support; carer-education/training versus conventional care or no support; multi-faceted/dimensional strategies versus conventional care or no support.[54] The review found that the evidence was inconclusive and the authors concluded that given the diversity of interventions aimed at supporting carers, the scale of Alzheimer's disease and the costs associated with providing support, further research is needed to adequately quantify any benefits.

2. Have their own written care plan which is given to them and implemented in discussion with them

No systematic reviews have been undertaken in this area.

Table 6. Details of systematic reviews relevant to NSF standard six*

	Study details	Intervention	Primary outcomes	Results	Quality score[#]	Comments
Family interventions	Cuijpers 1999[51]	Family interventions for carers of people with a mental illness	Relatives' burden of care	Compared with control, family interventions: ↓[a] relatives' burden	4	*Comments on review:* Only two databases searched *Comments on primary studies:* 16 RCTs and controlled studies (n=not stated) Diverse measures of relative's burden in included studies.
Respite care	Flint 1995[52]	Respite care	Caregivers burden and stress, psychiatric status, physical health and attitudes toward the patient; the dementia patient's cognition, behaviour, physical health and functioning	Compared with control, respite care: ↔[b] relatives' burden ↓[b] relationship between patient and relative ↔[b] carer's psychological health ↔[b] carer's physical health	4	*Comments on review:* Literature search limited to English language articles *Comments on primary studies:* 4 controlled trials (n=762). Lack of standardised criteria to make the diagnosis. Use of more than one type of respite care intervention. Use of respite service outside study by control groups
	McNally 1999[53]	Respite care	Carers' well-being including psychological well-being, carer stress or carer burden, and physical health	Compared with control, respite care: ↔[b] carer's well-being	4	*Comments on review:* No formal quality assessment of included studies. *Comments on primary studies:* 29 controlled and uncontrolled studies (n=2865) Majority of the primary studies were methodologically poor
Other interventions	Thompson 1998*[54]	Interventions provided by health and/or social services for carers of people with dementia	Carer's quality of life and/or physical health as measured by validated indicators	Inconclusive evidence	5	*Comments on review:* Limited search terms used. *Comments on primary studies:* 6 RCTs (n=> 301) Heterogeneous interventions with multiple outcomes and measures used. Small, relatively poor quality studies.

* For Cochrane reviews, year review was last updated
[#] Adapted from Oxman et al [9]. 1= extensive flaws, 7= minimal flaws in the review
↓ decrease in outcome as compared with standard care/comparison intervention.
↑ increase in outcome as compared with standard care/comparison intervention
↔ no difference in outcome between groups, or insufficient data to detect a difference
[a] results from pooled meta-analysis. Results significant at $p<0.05$
[b] results from narrative synthesis of results. Meta-analysis not performed due to clinical or statistical heterogeneity

Further details of these reviews are provided in Appendix 3.

5. NSF STANDARD SEVEN: PREVENTING SUICIDE

> Local health and social care communities should prevent suicide by implementing some or all of the previous standards, and in addition:
> 1. Support local prison staff in preventing suicides among prisoners
> 2. Ensure that staff are competent to assess the risk of suicide among individuals at greatest risk
> 3. Develop local systems for suicide audit to learn lessons and take any necessary action

Four reviews were included in this section.

1. Support for local prison staff in preventing suicides among prisoners
No systematic reviews of preventing suicide in prison have been undertaken.

2. Ensuring that staff are competent to assess the risk of suicide among individuals at greatest risk
One systematic review evaluated the effectiveness of objective personality assessment instruments in predicting suicidal intention.[55] These instruments included the California Personality Inventory; Edwards Preference Schedule; Eysenck Personality Tests; Millon Clinical Multiaxial Inventory (I-III); Minnesota Multiphasic Personality Inventory (1-2); Myers-Briggs Type Indicator; 16 Personality Factor Test; Neuroticism, Extroversion, Openness Personality Inventory; Personality Diagnostic Questionnaire. The review reported that there was scant evidence for most of the scales and lack of evidence for predictive utility on the part of the inventories reviewed.

3. Develop local systems for suicide audit to learn lessons and take any necessary action
No systematic reviews have been undertaken in the audit of suicide. It is, however, worth noting that there is a national confidential inquiry into suicide and homicide by people with mental illness.[92] Statistics on social and clinical characteristics of suicide as well as methods of suicide are collected.

Three reviews evaluated interventions to reduce the rate of repeated self-harm and the risk of suicide.[56-58] All three reviews focused primarily on therapeutic interventions. The Cochrane review also included studies that evaluated intensive intervention plus outreach; and emergency cards with which they either had 24-hour access to emergency advice from a psychiatrist, or could admit themselves to hospital. The review concluded that there still remains considerable uncertainty about which forms of psychosocial and physical treatments of self-harm patients are most effective. This review was also published in a journal and also formed the basis of an Effective Health Care Bulletin.[56, 59] Another review included studies of guaranteed in-patient shelters and psychosocial crisis interventions.[58] The review found that there was no clear evidence for a reduction in repeated suicide attempts with interventions which seek to increase compliance with aftercare, or which guarantee in-patient shelter in the event of an emergency or psychosocial crisis. The third review included evaluations of different settings of care, such as home versus outpatient treatment and inpatient versus outpatient psychotherapy.[57] It was of poor quality, but also reported that no suicide prevention strategies have been conclusively demonstrated to be effective

Areas not covered by systematic reviews include:
- self-harm intervention services
- supporting local prison staff in preventing suicide among prisoners
- developing local systems for suicide audit
- assertive outreach linked to court diversion.

Table 7. Details of systematic reviews relevant to NSF seven*

	Study details	Intervention	Primary outcomes	Results	Quality score[#]	Comments
Assessing the risk of suicide	Johnson 1999[55]	Prediction of suicidal intention using objective personality assessment instruments	Prediction of suicidal intention	↔[b] predictive value	3	*Comments on review*: Only one database searched for English language trials. No quality assessment of included studies. *Comments on primary studies*: 42 studies (n=not stated). Marked heterogeneity in study design and poor evidence for most scales
Prevention of suicide and self-harm	Hawton 1999*[56]	Problem solving; intensive intervention plus outreach; emergency card	Rate of repeated self-harm (fatal and non-fatal) within a follow-up period of up to 2 years	For all interventions: ↔[a] Trend towards reduced repetition of deliberate self-harm (not significant)	7	*Comments on review*: Methodologically sound *Comments on primary studies*: 23 RCTs (n=3014)
	Repper 1999[57]	Suicide prevention interventions	Reduction in deliberate self-harm and reduction in the risk of suicide	↔[b] No suicide prevention strategies have been conclusively demonstrated to be effective	3	*Comments on review*: Only included English language studies/reviews since 1990. No quality assessment, unclear inclusion/exclusion criteria. *Comments on primary studies*: 7 RCTs (n=1,290)
	Van der Sande 1997[58]	Psychosocial/ psychotherapeutic interventions	Incidence of repeated suicide attempts	Compared with control, guaranteed in-patient shelter: ↔[a] repeated suicide attempts	6	*Comments on review*: Search limited to English language literature *Comments on primary studies*: 15 RCTs (n=2019)

[#] Adapted from Oxman et al [9]. 1= extensive flaws, 7= minimal flaws in the review
* For Cochrane reviews, year review was last updated
↓ decrease in outcome as compared with standard care/comparison intervention.
↑ increase in outcome as compared with standard care/comparison intervention
↔ no difference in outcome between groups, or insufficient data to detect a difference
[a] results from pooled meta-analysis. Results significant at p<0.05
[b] results from narrative synthesis of results. Meta-analysis not performed due to clinical or statistical heterogeneity

Box 2.
Summary of areas where systematic reviews in mental health service delivery have been undertaken

NSF standard 1: Mental health promotion
- Mental health promotion for the general population and high risk groups

NSF standards 2 and 3: Primary care
- Primary or community care professionals in A&E departments
- Referral from primary to secondary care
- On-site mental health workers
- Improving primary prevention
- Recognition and/or management of mental disorders
- Setting of care for anorexia nervosa and depression
- Professional and/or social support for women with post-natal depression
- Interventions intended to affect adherence with prescribed, self-administered medications

NSF standards 4 and 5: People with a severe mental illness
- Prediction of imminent violence
- Community mental health teams and community mental health nurses
- Home based care (including ACT, case/care management/CPA, multidisciplinary teams, crisis intervention, assertive community therapy)
- Interventions for people with a dual diagnosis
- Patient-held information
- Supported employment and vocational rehabilitation
- Supported housing
- Day care and day hospitals
- Prompts to encouraging appointment attendance
- Planned short stay/brief admission to hospital
- Interventions for mentally disordered offenders

NSF standard 6: Caring for carers
- Family interventions
- Interventions for carers of people with dementia (including respite care, individualised service assessment and planning, technology-based networking, carer-education/training and multi-faceted/dimensional interventions)

NSF standard 7: Prevention of suicide
- Objective personality assessment instruments to predict suicidal intentions
- Suicide prevention interventions including intensive intervention plus outreach; and emergency cards with which people either had 24-hour access to emergency advice from a psychiatrist, or could admit themselves to hospital

Box 3.
Summary of areas where systematic reviews in mental health service delivery should be considered

NSF standard 1: Mental health promotion
- Reducing stigma and combating discrimination/social exclusion
- Increasing public awareness and understanding of mental health and mental illness

NSF standards 2 and 3: Primary care
- Further reviews of diagnosis and assessment of mental illness
- Generic approaches to managing prescribing in primary care
- Liaison psychiatrists/other mental health professionals in primary care settings
- Case management of depression by clinical pharmacists in a primary care setting
- 24 hour services and telephone helplines
- Primary care therapy teams and audit of psychological therapy services
- One stop shop clinics
- Self-help and self-help groups

NSF standards 4 and 5: People with a severe mental illness
- Twenty-four hour care
- Further reviews of community care package/setting of care interventions
- Hospital-based interventions such as: therapies within residential units or hospital wards (e.g. homelike social environment); crisis hospitalisation vs. short-term hospitalisation; scheduled intermittent or long-term hospitalisation; rapid discharge programme; custodial treatment
- Management issues such as: capitated integrated service agencies (ISAS); fee for service programmes; housing subsidies
- Patient interventions such as: therapeutic alliance; psychiatrist vs. GP
- Early interventions for people with schizophrenia
- Intensive 24-hour staffed residential and nursing homes
- Integrated health and social care management
- General practice registers for people with severe and enduring mental illness
- Culturally sensitive support
- Service user support
- Assessment and access to services for those coming into contact with the criminal justice system

NSF standard 6: Caring for carers
- Interventions aimed at carers of people with mental health
- Written care plans and needs assessment
- Checklists for GPs and primary care teams to help carers

NSF standard 7: Prevention of suicide
- Self-harm intervention services
- Supporting local prison staff in preventing suicide among prisoners
- Developing local systems for suicide audit
- Assertive outreach linked to court diversion

DISCUSSION
1. The evidence for the effectiveness of mental health service delivery interventions and links with the NSF Framework for mental health

Thirty-six completed systematic reviews and eight Cochrane protocols were included in this scoping review. Of the thirty-six reviews, nine were included in the NSF.[2,19,24,27,30,34,50,59,60] This disparity may be due to the different search strategies used (the search strategy for the NSF was not described), the different objectives of the two documents and the fact that some reviews have been published since the NSF.

NSF Standard 1: Mental Health Promotion

Mental health promotion was very difficult to define. Only one review, which specifically evaluated mental health promotion, was identified.[10] As the outcome of interest in this area is often mental health and well-being, a range of environmental and social interventions as well as traditional health promotion interventions could be included in this section. Searching for all possible systematic reviews, however, was beyond the resources available for this scoping review. Details of other systematic reviews that could fall under NSF standard one can be found in a document which contains a report on the national contract on mental health.[11] Areas not covered by systematic reviews include interventions to increase awareness and reduce the stigma of mental illness.

NSF Standards 2 and 3: Primary Care and Access to Services

Seven systematic reviews and two protocols were identified. Three systematic reviews (two in the protocol stage) evaluated interventions to improve the organisation of primary care services.[16-18] Two of these were on interventions aimed at the general population rather than specifically targeting people with mental health problems, but include/will include relevant studies. Two reviews evaluated interventions targeted at more accurate diagnosis and prevention.[12,13] There are still gaps in this area, however, where systematic reviews have not been undertaken. Three reviews evaluated interventions for people with a specific mental illness.[19,20,23] Two of these (one Cochrane protocol and one completed review) evaluated/will evaluate the setting of therapeutic interventions for anorexia nervosa and major depression, and the third evaluated professional and/or social support for women with postnatal depression. Finally, one review evaluated interventions intended to affect adherence with prescribed, self-administered medications.[21] There are still gaps in the area of primary care, however, where systematic reviews have not been undertaken (box 3). Although the NSF recommends round the clock contact with the local services and the use of NHS direct, neither have been evaluated in systematic reviews. However, such interventions may be difficult to evaluate in systematic reviews

NSF standards 4 and 5: Effective services for people with severe mental illness

Twenty-one systematic reviews and five protocols were identified. The care programme approach is standard care in the UK and many of the recommendations for care of people with severe mental illnesses in the NSF are based on such an approach. Overall, the included reviews concluded that ACT is an effective approach, and the care programme approach is less so. The NSF does, however, outline a national milestone, which is to have assertive outreach in place for service users on enhanced CPA and at risk of losing contact with services. A further national milestone in the NSF is to increase the percentage of community mental health teams and the evidence from a Cochrane review[24] suggest that this is an effective intervention.

One review evaluated crisis management,[34] but no reviews have evaluated the effectiveness of the range of 24-hour services. However, such interventions will be difficult to evaluate (see Appendix 4). A number of good reviews exist on the effectiveness of specific services that provide 24-hour care. Further reviews of other specific services that provide 24-hour care may be considered after prudent prioritisation. In deciding which studies to review, it is necessary to prioritise, focus research questions and establish appropriate comparisons. In doing so, it is important to evaluate specific types of services. It would be necessary to decide whether to evaluate the components of 24-hours services (e.g. to establish whether a 24-hour helpline is more effective than a daytime helpline) or the methods of gaining access to the services (e.g. to estimate the effectiveness of a telephone helpline in making 24-hour services accessible to people).

Only one systematic review considered care within the hospital setting and concluded that short stay was more effective than long stay or standard care.[36] No systematic reviews have been undertaken to evaluate interventions within the hospital setting such as home-like social environments. A series of four CRD reports[41-43,61] (two included in this paper) were designed to lay out the state of the current literature on mentally disordered offenders. The majority of the primary research, however, was for people with personality disorders.

NSF standards 6: Caring about carers
Four reviews were included in this section,[51-54] but only one included carers of people with a mental illness.[51] Although the needs of carers of people with dementia may be similar to those of people caring for someone with a mental illness, they were of lower quality than other reviews. Therefore, there is a need for further high quality systematic reviews to be undertaken in this area.

NSF standard 7: Preventing suicide
One systematic review evaluated the effectiveness of objective personality assessment instruments in predicting suicidal intention.[55] No other systematic reviews have been undertaken of risk assessment to self and/or others. Three other reviews primarily evaluated therapeutic interventions to reduce the rate of repeated self-harm and the risk of suicide.[56-58] One of the national milestones of the NSF is for A&E departments to develop and implement protocols for those who present with self-harm. There are no systematic reviews specifically evaluating which protocols would be effective, but a Cochrane review is underway to evaluate primary and community health care professionals in hospital emergency departments and it may include relevant trials.[17] No systematic reviews evaluating interventions to support local prison staff in preventing suicides among prisoners have been undertaken.

2. Strengths and weaknesses of the systematic reviews
The quality of all the reviews included was scored using criteria adapted from a checklist for review articles.[9] Cochrane reviews in general scored higher then the non-Cochrane reviews and were published more recently. They are regularly updated and so will incorporate new evidence, as it becomes available. Furthermore the medium in which the are prepared and published (electronically) means that they can be modified to include, for example, information on additional outcomes that are deemed to be important. However, some Cochrane reviews have not been updated recently because of lack of resources.[2,30]

Although areas covered by systematic reviews are outlined in the above section, some of the reviews did not include outcomes such as user's social networks, user and carer satisfaction, social relationships and quality of life. That is, they lacked a consumer perspective. Such outcomes were assessed more frequently in Cochrane reviews than in non-Cochrane reviews.

As well as summarising evidence on clinical effectiveness, systematic reviews also have the potential to inform economic and policy evaluations.[62] There are, however, some limitations of systematic reviews. Most importantly, if the studies in the review are of poor quality, or do not measure appropriate outcomes, systematic reviews cannot overcome these limitations. In some cases (such as the review of life skills programmes for chronic mental illnesses)[47] there may be few included studies, even though a thorough search of the literature has been undertaken. Thus the ability to draw conclusions may be severely limited. Systematic reviews can, however, identify the gaps in the evidence from primary research and make recommendations for further research. For example, the Cochrane review of interventions of people with dual disorders found the quality of design and reporting of the six relevant trials (four of which were small with only 29-42 participants) was quite low.[39] The review recommended that further trials of specialist integrated programmes are urgently needed before they are adopted more widely.

In order to minimise bias, many systematic reviews only include RCTs. Whilst they are the best evidence to evaluate the effectiveness of interventions, other evidence from sources such as non-randomised or qualitative studies may increase the relevance of the findings of a review. The NSF synthesises five types of evidence which includes systematic reviews, randomised controlled trials, well designed intervention studies without randomisation, well designed observational studies, and expert opinion (including the opinion of service users and carers).

3. Generalisability of results

A further problem is that the results of a systematic review may not be generalisable to the UK setting. For example, many of the trials of ACT were undertaken in the USA. Whilst the intervention (ACT) may in principle be the same as in the UK, the comparison group (standard care) may differ between countries. Thus, ACT may be more or less effective in the UK depending on what the standard care is. Furthermore, the local system in which ACT operates in the UK may be important as high fidelity ACT may founder if not part of a coherent system of care. The Cochrane review of ACT recommended that there may be a stronger case for further ACT versus standard care comparisons in countries outside the USA, particularly those with highly developed primary care services, such as the UK.[30] It would also be advisable to standardise standard care as much as possible so that we know what is compared to what. In addition, more energy should be invested to measure the success of implementation of these interventions (compare this to compliance measurement in studies on drugs).

4. Limitations of the scoping review

Due to the remit of this scoping review, a distinction had to be made between service delivery interventions (which were included) and therapeutic interventions (which were excluded). However, it was often difficult to distinguish between what is therapeutic and what is health service. Thus there is a potential that some therapeutic interventions which evaluated the setting of care may have been missed. An example would be all the reviews on depression management in primary care not identified by the review, which, although about therapy, could include a lot about issues relevant to the setting as well. Furthermore, by making this distinction, it may be, for example that what health professionals are doing therapeutically in ACT is the crucial variable when comparing this to standard care or to case management. Pure clinical research tends to ignore health service interventions just as health service research ignores therapies. Psychosocial interventions (e.g. problem solving therapy) were excluded in our review yet these are now being perceived as bordering with service delivery.

Identifying all of the areas where there have been no systematic reviews was difficult. The Advisory Board gave input into areas that had not been fully evaluated, and the topic lists from relevant Cochrane Review Groups such as the Schizophrenia Group were scrutinised, as well as examples of good practice outlined in the NSF. However, it may be that there are further gaps that have not been identified.

It is recognised that not all questions relating to mental health service delivery can be answered by systematic reviews, as the majority of research in this area is medically orientated. There is also a need for 'people-orientated' research on the success of various interventions. Arguably the majority of mental health care takes place not only outside the psychiatric system but also outside health and social-care all together. For example, support may be provided by the 'community', family, friends, and/or neighbours. Therefore, in order to comprehensively review the costs and other effectiveness of mental health services a way needs to be found to measure the input from the informal care sector and the social/environment (occupation, accommodation).

CONCLUSIONS

Thirty-six good quality systematic reviews have been undertaken and eight are being prepared in the areas of mental health promotion and mental health service delivery. Few of the systematic reviews, however, were able to conclude that an intervention was effective or not. This was due primarily to the poor quality, or limited amount of primary research. The only two interventions which could be considered to be effective from the included primary research were assertive outreach and community mental health teams. The care programme approach was not considered to be an effective intervention. For all of the other areas of mental health service delivery evaluated by the systematic reviews, interventions have been evaluated poorly, (or not at all) in the primary research.

There are still many areas of mental health service delivery interventions which have not been evaluated by systematic reviews including services targeting more accurate diagnosis and assessment of common mental health problems; interventions within hospital settings, 24-hour staffed accommodation; more accurate assessment of risk of imminent violence (to self or others), and interventions for carers of people with a mental health problem. Only some included outcomes such as user's social networks, user and carer satisfaction, social relationships and quality of life. These outcomes should be incorporated into future systematic reviews and primary research. Undertaking systematic reviews in these areas will not only help to inform about what evidence is available, but can make recommendations for future primary research. It is recommended that Cochrane reviews should be undertaken where possible, but resources need to be available to keep them up-to-date.

PART 2. COST-EFFECTIVENESS OF MENTAL HEALTH SERVICE DELIVERY INTERVENTIONS

BACKGROUND

The Department of Health (DOH) commissioned the NHS Centre for Reviews and Dissemination (NHS CRD) to undertake a review of evidence on the cost-effectiveness of the provision of mental health care services, based on the seven standards of the National Service Framework for Mental Health.

AIM

To undertake a literature review of economic evaluations of mental health service interventions.

OBJECTIVES

To identify and assess the cost-effectiveness evidence from full economic evaluations of different modes of providing mental health services

INCLUSION CRITERIA

All studies considered in this literature review had to meet the following inclusion criteria for methodology, interventions and participants:

1. Methodology of included studies

Inclusion Criteria
- All studies of cost-effectiveness, cost utility or cost-benefit.

Exclusion Criteria
- Methodological papers, discursive analysis of costs/benefits, partial evaluation studies

2. Interventions evaluated in the studies

Inclusion Criteria
- Mental health promotion
- Mental health service delivery/organisational interventions
- Different settings (e.g. inpatient vs outpatient) or methods of delivery (e.g. nurse vs doctor) for a therapeutic intervention

Exclusion Criteria
- Therapeutic interventions aimed at the individual, such as pharmacological or psychological therapies.

3. Participants included in the studies

Inclusion Criteria
- Adults aged 16 - 65 years with a mental health problem
- For economic evaluations of mental health promotion interventions, subjects were the general adult population, some of whom may be at risk of developing mental health problems
- People with a dual diagnosis (e.g. drug misuse and a mental illness)
- Carers of people with a mental health problem
- Carers of people with dementia (may be generalisable to other carers)

Exclusion Criteria
- Children, adolescents or people over 65 years of age
- People who abuse alcohol or drugs, unless the people also have a mental health problem (i.e. dual diagnosis)
- People with mental disabilities such as Down's Syndrome
- Sex offenders
- People with a personality disorder

SEARCH STRATEGY
Due to the limited time frame for the report, the NHS Economic Evaluation Database (NHS-EED) was the only source of economic evaluations. This database identifies studies from three databases: Current Contents-Clinical Medicine (1994 onwards), MEDLINE (1995 onwards) and CINAHL (1995 onwards). It also includes papers identified from handsearching the major biomedical journals and working papers from research centres specialising in health economics. Studies in NHS-EED are not selected for inclusion on the basis of their quality, but trained abstractors comment on the quality of the study and other relevant issues. A search strategy for the database was developed by an information specialist (KW) to identify all full economic evaluations of the delivery of mental health services (see Appendix 5.)

Data extraction:
Two reviewers (RJ and ZDB) independently screened studies that met inclusion criteria, checking disagreements with a third reviewer (GtR). Relevant sections from NHS-EED abstractions were tabulated. Studies identified by experts (Sarah Byford and Jennifer Beecham) were extracted. The quality of these additional studies was <u>not</u> assessed.

RESULTS
The search resulted in a total of 467 hits, of which 21 studies met our inclusion criteria and were abstracted. A further six studies were identified after discussion with an expert, bringing the total to 28 studies.[63-89] These studies were grouped using the objectives of the National Service Framework (NSF) standards. Full details of the included studies can be found in Appendix 6.

Eleven of the studies were undertaken in the USA or Canada, 13 in the UK, two in the Netherlands and one in Australia. Studies were conducted between 1980 and 2000, with the majority (83%) being published in 1995 or after. Twenty of the studies were RCTs, four were non-RCTs and the rest were cohort, cross-sectional or before-after studies.

Eighteen studies evaluated the cost-effectiveness of interventions in patients with a severe mental illness, eight evaluated interventions in primary care, and one evaluated interventions for carers of people with dementia. These studies are described more fully under the relevant NSF standards.

NSF STANDARD ONE: MENTAL HEALTH PROMOTION
No economic evaluations evaluating mental health promotion interventions were identified.

NSF STANDARDS TWO AND THREE: PRIMARY CARE AND ACCESS TO SERVICES
Eight studies evaluated the cost effectiveness of interventions in the primary care setting (see table 8). Five were undertaken in the UK and three in the USA.

Community care vs hospital or GP care
Five studies (four UK and one US based) evaluated the cost-effectiveness of community interventions for people with non-psychotic mental illnesses such as anxiety or depression.[72,73,79,81,86] Follow-ups varied from 3 to 18 months. Four out of the five reported that community care was more cost-effective than hospital or GP care. The fifth study would also have found the community intervention to be the most cost-effective strategy if the economic analysis had been based on both direct and indirect costs.[73]

Limitations of studies
Most of the studies were of reasonable quality, but the sample size was less than 100 in four out of five of them. Of the four studies that found community care to be cost-effective, one trial only reported cost-effectiveness for a sub-group.[86] Given the small numbers, this sub-group analysis should be interpreted with caution. One study was a non-RCT and because of the lack of randomisation, sensitivity analysis, and statistical analysis of the costs, the results of this study also need to be treated with some caution.[72] Costs were limited to NHS costs.

Table 8. NSF standards 2 & 3: details of economic evaluation studies

Study details	Design	Participants	Intervention	Control	Intervention more effective than control?	Intervention cheaper than control?	Intervention Cost-effective?
Community care vs hospital or GP care							
Goldberg 1996 [72] UK	CCT N=60 FU= 6 months	People with depression or anxiety	Community-based team	Hospital service	No difference in clinical outcomes	Yes	Yes¶
Gournay 1995 [73] UK	RCT N=177 FU= 24 weeks	People with non psychotic conditions	Psychiatric nurse (CPN)	Continuing GP care	No difference	Yes	Yes¶
Mangen 1983 [79] UK	RCT N=71 FU = 18 months	People with neurosis, affective psychosis	Community psychiatric nurse (CPN)	Outpatient psychiatric care	Yes for consumer satisfaction. No difference in symptom severity or family burden.	Yes	Yes¶
Merson 1996 [81] UK	RCT N= 100 FU= 3 months	Psychiatric A&E attenders	Early intervention community service	District hospital service	No difference	Yes	Yes
Von Korff 1998 [86] USA	RCT N=74 FU= 1 year	People with depression	Collaborative care in primary setting	Usual care	Yes for major depression	No	Yes for major but not minor depression¶
GP training and guidelines vs control							
Morriss 1998 [82] UK	CBA N=215 FU=3 months	People with somatising disorders	GP training package	No training	Yes, more people were successfully treated following GP training	Yes Total costs pre-training: £34,135; Post-training: £28,913	Yes Marginal cost-effectiveness ratio £325¶
Smith 1995 [83] USA	RCT N=56 FU= 2 years	People with somatising disorders	GP guidelines	No guidelines	Yes, improved physical functioning	Yes	Yes¶
Short stay units vs long stay units							
Fontana 1997 [69] USA	CCT N=785 FU = 1 year	People with post traumatic stress disorder (PTSD)	Short-stay PTSD unit	Long-term inpatient PTSD unit	Yes, greater improvement for symptoms and alcohol abuse	Yes	Unclear

RCT: randomised controlled trial; **CCT**: controlled clinical trial **CBA**: controlled before and after study; **FU**: follow up; **CPN**: community psychiatric nurse; ¶ NHS-EED did not provide enough details on either the perspective of the analysis (NHS or societal), the results for all measured outcomes or the statistical precision of the cost estimates to draw a definitive conclusion. Consult the last three columns of the appendix for more details.

GP guidelines and training

Two studies, one undertaken in the UK[82] and one undertaken in the USA[83] examined the cost-effectiveness of training GPs or providing guidelines for treating primary care somatising patients. Both were found to be cost-effective compared with standard care.

Limitations of studies

Both studies had limitations and thus conclusions should be treated with caution. One study[82] used a before-after design, which does not control for the natural time trend and Hawthorne effects. In addition, the lack of sensitivity analyses and details on patient characteristics further limit the applicability of the findings. The other study[83] has three drawbacks. First, it is small. Second, it exaggerates its precision by analysing at the patient level while randomising at the physician level. Finally, it uses charges instead of costs.

Table 9. NSF standards 4 and 5: details of economic evaluation studies of community care vs in-patient hospital care

Study details	Design	Participants	Intervention	Control	Intervention more effective than control?	Intervention cheaper than control?	Intervention cost-effective?
Van Minnen 1997[85] Netherlands	RCT N=50 FU=28 weeks	People with severe mental illness and mental retardation	Outreach treatment	In-patient hospital treatment	No significant difference in psychiatric symptoms	Yes, outreach costs were 40% lower than hospital treatment	Yes¶
Creed 1997[66] UK	RCT N=187 FU=12 months	Moderately ill people with schizophrenia, depression or neurosis	Day hospital treatment	In-patient hospital treatment	Clinical and social outcomes were similar, except for two	Yes, cheaper for direct costs but may be more costly for carers	Yes¶
Wiersma 1995[88] Netherlands	RCT N=103 FU=2 years	People with a severe mental illness	Day treatment with community care	In-patient hospital treatment	Yes for increased compliance/self-care. No for health service use	No significant difference	Yes¶
Hyde 1987[76] UK	RCT N=22 FU=2 years	Psychiatric inpatients	Hostel ward	In-patient hospital psychiatric unit	Yes in social outcomes, but no in clinical outcomes	Yes, less hotel costs	Yes¶
Beecham 1996[63] UK	Cohort N=133 FU=12 months	Psychiatric inpatients	Community care (accommodation)	In-patient hospital treatment	No significant difference in most outcomes. Small improvement in depression.	Yes, average cost of week was £268 less expensive	Yes¶
Hawthorne 1999[75] USA	CCT N=518 FU=4 months	Psychiatric inpatients	Short-term residential treatment	In-patient hospital treatment	No difference in most outcomes	Yes, the intervention was cheaper	Yes¶
Weisbrod 1980[87] USA	CCT N=not stated FU=3 years	Mental disorder	Community-based intervention, "Training in Community Living".	In-patient hospital treatment	Yes, less symptoms and more satisfaction	Not for health services but yes for society.	Yes¶

RCT: randomised controlled trial; **CCT**: controlled clinical trial; **FU**: follow up; **CE**: cost effectiveness; ¶ NHS-EED did not provide enough details on either the perspective of the analysis (NHS or societal), the results for all measured outcomes or the statistical precision of the cost estimates to draw a definitive conclusion. Consult the last three columns of the appendix for more details.

Short stay units vs long stay units

One study estimated the cost-effectiveness of long-term specialised inpatient post-traumatic stress disorder (PTSD) units, relative to short-stay specialised PTSD units and to non-specialised general psychiatric units for the treatment of PTSD in Vietnam War veterans.[69] A formal synthesis of costs and benefits was not performed, but the authors reported that long-stay inpatient PTSD units are costly, relative to short-stay specialised evaluation and brief treatment PTSD units and general psychiatric units. Because of several limitations of the study, the authors' conclusions, that a move to short stay inpatient units is cost effective within the study setting, are not justified by the study findings.

NSF STANDARDS 4 AND 5: EFFECTIVE SERVICES FOR PEOPLE WITH SEVERE MENTAL ILLNESS

Eighteen studies evaluated the cost-effectiveness of interventions for people with a severe mental illness. Seven were undertaken in the UK, eight in the USA, two in The Netherlands and one in Australia.

Community care vs in-patient hospital care

Seven economic evaluations of community care compared with in-patient hospital care were identified (see table 9).[63,66,75,76,85,87,88] The types of interventions included one study of outreach treatment, two studies of day care or day hospitals, two studies of types of accommodation; one study of a community training programme and one study of short-term residential care. Overall, the majority reported that community interventions were more effective, or at least as effective as hospital care, and cheaper or no more expensive. The majority concluded that community care was a viable alternative to hospital care.

Limitations of studies

Sample size in two of the studies was 50 subjects or less, and for one study sample size was not stated[87] thus conclusions regarding effectiveness may not be justified due to an inadequate sample size. One study[88] had major problems in the analysis of costs (see appendix 1 for further details). Many important indirect costs were omitted, therefore cost results were assumptions and this study was hypothesis generating.

Comparisons of different types of community care

Eleven economic evaluations compared different types of community care (see table 10).[64,65,67,70,71,74,77,78,80,84,89] Two studies compared community multi-disciplinary teams with standard outpatient care, but reported conflicting results on effectiveness and costs.[71,84] A further study compared transitional case management with outpatient care and reported that the former was cost-effective.[64]

Two studies compared the cost-effectiveness of intensive case management with standard case management.[74,77] Both reported that intensive case management was neither more effective, nor less costly than standard case management.

Three economic evaluations of assertive community treatment (ACT) were undertaken.[65,78,89] Two compared ACT to standard case management, and another compared it to usual community services. The patient groups varied, with one study including only people with a dual diagnosis, and the other two including mentally ill homeless people. All studies found the standard care to be at least as cost-effective as the interventions.

Other community approaches

One study compared a community support team with community psychiatric nurse teams, but found no difference in costs or effectiveness.[80] Another study compared modified therapeutic community with standard care, and found it to be more effective in improving psychological function but more expensive. However this study did not perform a full economic analysis.[70] A third study evaluated community care in three different regions in the USA and found community-based care to be more cost-effective than hospital-based care.[67]

Limitations of the studies

Seven of these studies were undertaken outside the UK and thus generalisability to the UK setting may be limited. The study which compared three US regions was limited by its observational design, small sample size and insufficient details of cost estimation.[67]

Table 10. NSF standards 4 and 5: details of economic evaluation studies of different types of community care

Study details	Design	Participants	Intervention	Control	Intervention more effective than control?	Intervention cheaper than control?	Intervention cost-effective?
Community vs out-patient care							
Tyrer 1998[84] UK	RCT N=154 FU=1 year	People with a severe mental illness	Community multi-disciplinary team	Hospital-based care programme (outpatient)	No difference	Yes, was cheaper than control (average cost £16,765 vs £19,125)	Yes¶
Gater 1997[71] UK	RCT N=63 FU=4 years	Chronic schizophrenia	Community multi-disciplinary team	Hospital-based care programme (outpatient)	Yes, better quality care at 2 & 4 years	No significant differences	A synthesis of costs and benefits was not performed.
Chiverton 1999[64] USA	RCT N=243 FU=3 months	Psychiatric inpatients	Transitional case management (psychiatric nurses)	Traditional care (outpatient care)	Yes, more effective in reducing depression and hospital stay	Yes, saved $175,375 over the period of analysis	Yes¶
Intensive case management vs standard case management							
UK700 Group, 2000[74] UK	RCT N=667 FU=2 years	People with a severe mental illness	Intensive case management	Standard case management	No difference in hospital days or other outcomes.	No difference in average costs	No
Johnston 1998[77] Australia	RCT N=73 FU=12 months	Severely disabled people with mental illness	Intensive case management	Routine case management	No difference in clinical outcomes	No, more expensive than control ($28,895 vs $21,150)	No¶
Assertive community treatment vs standard case management or usual services							
Clark 1998[65] USA	RCT N=223 FU=3 years	People with severe mental disorder and substance use disorder	Assertive community treatment (ACT)	Standard case management	No significant difference	No significant difference	No¶
Wolff, 1997[89] USA	RCT N=85 FU=18 months	People with severe mental illness who were (or at risk of becoming) homeless	ACT or ACT with community workers	Brokerage case management	Yes, ACT resulted in greater reduction in symptoms, and satisfaction	No significant differences in cost	Yes¶
Lehman 1999[78] USA	RCT N=152 FU=not stated	Homeless persons with severe mental illness	Assertive community treatment (ACT)	Usual services	Significantly more outpatient visits, but significantly less in-patient days.	Yes, the overall average costs per ACT patient was $15 732 less	Perhaps. ACT was 45% more efficient. However, incremental CE ratio was not significant
Other community care approaches							
McCrone 1994[80] UK	RCT N=82 FU=18 months	People with severe mental illnesses	Community support team (CST)	Community psychiatric nurse teams (CPN)	No significant differences	Yes, total costs were an average of £110 less per week	No difference beyond the short term in costs or cost-effectiveness
French 1999[70] USA	Cohort N=281 FU=2 years	Homeless mentally ill	Modified therapeutic community	Standard care	Yes, more effective in improving psychological functioning.	No	Possible, but no cost-effectiveness analysis undertaken

Study details	Design	Participants	Intervention	Control	Intervention more effective than control?	Intervention cheaper than control?	Intervention cost-effective?
Dickey 1997[67] USA	Cross-sectional analysis of retrospective cohort N=144 FU=1 year	Psychiatric Medicaid beneficiaries	Community Care	Hospital-based care	No significant differences	Yes	Yes¶

RCT: randomised controlled trial; CCT: controlled clinical trial; FU: follow up; CE: cost effectiveness; ¶ NHS-EED did not provide enough details on either the perspective of the analysis (NHS or societal), the results for all measured outcomes or the statistical precision of the cost estimates to draw a definitive conclusion. Consult the last three columns of the appendix for more details.

NSF STANDARD 6: CARING FOR CARERS

One RCT looked at the cost-effectiveness of providing support to carers living with a relative with dementia but found no difference compared to community nursing (see table 11).[68] The study was limited by the small sample size and the large variance in the quality of life scores of carers.

Table 11. NSF standard 6: details of economic evaluation studies

Study details	Design	Participants	Intervention	Control	Intervention more effective than control?	Intervention cheaper than control?	Intervention cost-effective?
Drummond 1991[68] UK	RCT N=60 FU=6 months	Carers of people with dementia	Caregiver support programme	Conventional Community Care	No	No	No¶

¶ NHS-EED did not provide enough details on either the perspective of the analysis (NHS or societal), the results for all measured outcomes or the statistical precision of the cost estimates to draw a definitive conclusion. Consult the last three columns of the appendix for more details.

NSF STANDARD 7: PREVENTING SUICIDE

No economic evaluations evaluating interventions to prevent suicide were identified.

DISCUSSION

No economic evaluations related to NSF standards one and seven were found. This leaves three areas where studies have been undertaken: primary care and access to services (8 studies), services for people with severe mental illness (19 studies), and care for carers (1 study).

For a full economic evaluation to be flawless both the effectiveness and the costing components have to be of high quality. Therefore, it is very difficult to conduct a flawless full economic evaluation. It should come as no surprise that many studies reviewed here suffer from fairly severe validity problems. We strongly emphasise that these problems greatly restrict the applicability of the findings. In addition, from the NHS-EED data it was very often difficult to tell what perspective (NHS or societal) was taken in the analysis. As it may be relatively easy to transfer costs from the health care sector to the social sector the societal perspective seems preferable. Most evaluations reviewed here are based on single studies and many involved small sample sizes. In principle, small sample size would not be a problem if findings were statistically poolable. However, the prerequisites for pooling (between-study similarity of patients, interventions, and outcome measures) are not met. This means that all studies remain 'stand-alone' studies and small sample size then becomes a concern. The sample size requirements from the cost perspective are often more severe than for effectiveness, due to the skewed distribution commonly found with cost data. As indicated by the symbol (¶), the YES statements in the last columns of the tables in this document mostly refer to the position of the point estimates and do not necessarily imply a statistically significant difference at the conventional 5% level. Similarly, the NO statements do not necessarily imply a precise estimate near the point of 'no difference'.

Half of the studies were based outside the UK and thus may not be generalisable to the UK setting. Although recalculation of costs based on resource-use data, if available, may be possible, the effectiveness and resource-use data may still be inapplicable to the UK, given differences in service types, service availability, referral patterns and patient populations. The single effectiveness estimates may differ from those generated by combined estimates from systematic reviews. <u>When an economic modelling exercise is to be undertaken, it may be better to use effectiveness data from systematic reviews.</u> Many studies recruited patients from different diagnostic categories and the overall results from such studies may not reflect the true results for the component disease categories. Of course subgroup analyses may address this issue, but it is probably wiser to recruit prognostically homogeneous patient groups in single primary studies.

A particularly important issue in mental health services is the perspective taken for the cost calculations. Many studies take a healthcare sector perspective ignoring the potentially large costs and productivity losses incurred by patients, their carers and other statutory sectors, such as social services and the voluntary sector. <u>The reader is referred to the last column in the appendix for detailed comments on single studies as perceived by trained health economists working for the NHS-EED database.</u>

LIMITATIONS OF PRESENT REVIEW
The work reported here has its own limitations. The use of NHS-EED only does not guarantee full coverage of the literature. This choice was necessary given the strict time restraints imposed on the review team. NHS-EED does not cover PsycLIT and EMBASE, for example, and thus we cannot exclude the possibility that we missed some important studies. The fact that our advisers found six studies, which our searches had not picked up, may illustrate this. Working with the NHS-EED records as the main source of information, infrequently consulting the original papers made it even more difficult to get a clear picture of the patients included in the studies and the exact nature of the interventions used. Furthermore, none of the reviewers has had a firm training in health economics, which may have caused some oversights.

REFERENCES

1. CE, Rice K. Crisis intervention for people with severe mental illnesses. *Cochrane Database of Systematic Reviews. Issue 3.* Oxford: Update Software, 2000.

35. Henderson C, Laugharne R. Patient held clinical information for people with psychotic illnesses. *Cochrane Database of Systematic Reviews. Issue 3.* Oxford: Update Software, 2000. NHS Executive *National Service Framework for Mental Health*: London: Department of Health, 1999.

2. Marshall M, Gray A, Lockwood A, Green R. Case management for people with severe mental disorders. *Cochrane Database of Systematic Reviews. Issue 3.* Oxford: Update Software, 2000.

3. Burns T. Case management, care management and care programming. *British Journal of Psychiatry* 1997;170:393-395.

4. NHS CRD. Making cost-effectiveness information accessible: the NHS economic evaluation database Report 6. York: University of York. 1996.

5. Hayes AA, Macdonald GM. Supported housing for people with severe mental disorders. *Cochrane Database of Systematic Reviews. Issue 3.* Oxford: Update Software, 2000.

6. Department of Health. *Our healthier nation: a contract for health.* Wetherby: Stationery Office, 1998.

7. Department of Health. *Modernising Mental Health Services. Safe sound and supportive.* Wetherby: Stationery Office, 1998.

8. Jadad A, Cook D, Jones A, et al. Methodology and reports of systematic reviews and meta-analyses. A comparison of Cochrane Reviews with articles published in paper-based journals. *British Medical Journal* 1999;280:278 - 280.

9. Oxman A. Checklists for review articles. *British Medical Journal* 1994;309:648-51.

10. Tilford S, Delaney F, Vogels M. Effectiveness of mental health promotion interventions: a review. *Health Promotion Effectiveness Reviews* 1997;4:1-162.

11. Contributors to the Cochrane Collaboration and the Campbell Collaboration. Evidence from systematic reviews of research relevant to implementing the 'wider public health' agenda. York: NHS Centre for Reviews and Dissemination, 2000.

12. Kroenke K, Taylor-Vaisey A, Dietrich AJ, Oxman TE. Interventions to improve provider diagnosis and treatment of mental disorders in primary care - A critical review of the literature. *Psychosomatics* 2000;41:39-52.

13. Hulscher ME, Wensing M, Grol RP, van der Weijden T, van Weel C. Interventions to improve the delivery of preventive services in primary care. *American Journal of Public Health* 1999;89:737-746.

14. Hulscher M, Wensing M, Van der Weijden T, Grol R, Van Weel C. Interventions to implement prevention in primary care (protocol). *Cochrane Database of Systematic Reviews. Issue 3.* Oxford: Update Software, 2000.

15. Bower P, Sibbald B. On-site mental health workers in primary care: effects on professional practice. *Cochrane Database of Systematic Reviews. Issue 3.* Oxford: Update Software, 2000.

16. Bower P, Sibbald B. Systematic review of the effect of on-site mental health professionals on the clinical behaviour of general practitioners. *British Medical Journal* 2000;320:614-7.

17. Abi-Aad G, Johnson L, Mays N, Roberts E. Primary and community health care professionals in hospital emergency departments: effects on process and outcome of care and resources [protocol]. *Cochrane Database of Systematic Reviews. Issue 3.* Oxford: Update Software, 2000.

18. Grimshaw JM, Winkens RAG, Shirran L, et al. Interventions to improve physician referrals from primary to secondary care. *Cochrane Database of Systematic Reviews. Issue 3.* Oxford: Update Software, 2000.

19. Ray KL, Hodnett ED. Caregiver support for postpartum depression. *Cochrane Database of Systematic Reviews. Issue 3.* Oxford: Update Software, 2000.

20. Boyle P, Stimpson N, Lewis G, Farmer A. Interventions available for the treatment of anorexia nervosa specialist clinics versus non-specialist clinics. *Cochrane Database of Systematic Reviews. Issue 3.* Oxford: Update Software, 2000.

21. Haynes RB, Montague P, Oliver T, et al. Interventions for helping patients to follow prescriptions for medications. *Cochrane Database of Systematic Reviews. Issue 3.* Oxford: Update Software, 2000.

22. NHS CRD. The treatment of depression in primary care. *Effective Health Care* 1993;5.
23. Schulberg HC, Katon W, Simon GE, Rush AJ. Treating major depression in primary care practice - an update of the agency for health care policy and research practice guidelines. *Archives of General Psychiatry* 1998;55:1121-1127.
24. Tyrer P, Coid J, Simmonds S, Joseph P, Marriott S. Community mental health teams (CMHTs) for people with severe mental illnesses and disordered personality. *Cochrane Database of Systematic Reviews. Issue 3.* Oxford: Update Software, 2000.
25. Brooker C, Repper JM, Booth A. The effectiveness of community mental health nursing: a review. *Journal of Clinical Effectiveness* 1996;1:44-50.
26. Holloway F, Oliver N, Collins E, Carson J. Case management - a critical review of the outcome literature. *European Psychiatry* 1995;10:113-128.
27. Mueser KT, Bond GR, Drake RE, Resnick SG. Models of community care for severe mental illness: a review of research on case management. *Schizophrenia Bulletin* 1998;24:37-74.
28. Wadhwa S, Lavizzo-Mourey R. Do innovative models of health care delivery improve quality of care for selected vulnerable populations? a systematic review. *Journal on Quality Improvement* 1999;25:408-421.
29. Scott JE, Dixon LB. Assertive community treatment and case management for schizophrenia. *Schizophrenia-Bulletin* 1995;21:657-668.
30. Marshall M, Lockwood A. Assertive community treatment for people with severe mental disorders. *Cochrane Database of Systematic Reviews. Issue 3.* Oxford: Update Software, 2000.
31. Latimer EA. Economic impacts of assertive community treatment: a review of the literature (review). *Canadian Journal of Psychiatry - Revue Canadienne de Psychiatrie* 1999;44:443-454.
32. Mueser KT, Drake RE, Bond GR. Recent advances in psychiatric rehabilitation for patients with severe mental illness. (Review) (213 refs). *Harvard Review of Psychiatry* 1997;5:123-37.
33. Burns T. A systematic review of home treatment compared with admission for mental health problems evaluated in terms of clinical, social, and cost outcomes, user and carer acceptability and sustainability of programmes. *Unpublished HTA monograph,* 2000.
34. Joy CB, Adams
36. Johnstone P, Zolese G. Systematic review of the effectiveness of planned short hospital stays for mental health care. *British Medical Journal* 1999;318:1387-90.
37. Cally J, Burns T, Cornas A. Day centres for severe mental Illness. *Cochrane Database of Systematic Reviews. Issue 3.* Oxford: Update Software, 2000.
38. Wing, J., Marriott, S., Palmer, C. and Thomas, V. Management of imminent violence: clinical practice guidelines to support mental health services. *Occasional Paper OP41.* London: Royal College of Psychiatrists, 1998
39. Ley A, Jeffery DP, McLaren S, Siegfried N. Treatment programmes for people with both severe mental illness and substance misuse. *Cochrane Database of Systematic Reviews. Issue 3.* Oxford: Update Software, 2000.
40. Drake RE, Mercer-McFadden C, Mueser KT, McHugo GJ, Bond GR. Review of integrated mental health and substance abuse treatment for patients with dual disorders. *Schizophrenia Bulletin* 1998;24:589-608.
41. Lart R, Payne S, Beaumont B, Macdonald G, Mistry T. Women and secure psychiatric services: a literature review. *CRD Report 14,* 1999;14:1-102.
42. Lees J, Manning N, Rawlings B. Therapeutic community effectiveness: a systematic international review of therapeutic community treatment for people with personality disorders and mentally disordered offenders. *CRD Report 17,* York, NHS Centre for Reviews and Disemmintation 1999;17:1-214.
43. Hagell A, Dourke Dowling S. Scoping review of literature on the health and care of mentally disordered offenders. *CRD Report 16,* 1999;16.
44. Bond GR, Drake RE, Mueser KT, Becker DR. An update on supported employment for people with severe mental Illness (review). *Psychiatric Services* 1997;48:335-346.
45. Lehman AF. Vocational rehabilitation in schizophrenia. *Schizophrenia Bulletin* 1995;21:645-56.
46. Crowther R, Bond G, Huxley P, Marshall M. Vocational rehabilitation for people with severe mental disorders. *Cochrane Database of Systematic Reviews. Issue 3.* Oxford: Update Software, 2000.

47. Nicol MM, Robertson L, Connaughton JA. Life skills programmes for chronic mental illnesses. *Cochrane Database of Systematic Reviews. Issue 3.* Oxford: Update Software, 2000.

48. Almaraz-Serrano AM, Marshall M, Creed F. Day hospitals for people with psychiatric disorders. *Cochrane Database of Systematic Reviews. Issue 3.* Oxford: Update Software, 2000.

49. Reda S, Makhoul S. Prompts to encourage appointment attendance for people with severe mental illness. *Cochrane Database of Systematic Reviews. Issue 3.* Oxford: Update Software, 2000.

50. Johnstone P, Zolese G. Length of hospitalisation for people with severe mental illness. *Cochrane Database of Systematic Reviews. Issue 3.* Oxford: Update Software, 2000.

51. Cuijpers P. The effects of family interventions on relatives' burden: a meta-analysis. *Journal of Mental Health* 1999;8:275-85.

52. Flint AJ. Effects of respite care on patients with dementia and their caregivers. *International Psychogeriatrics* 1995;7:505-517.

53. McNally S, Ben Shlomo Y, Newman S. The effects of respite care on informal carers' well-being: A systematic review. *Disability-and-Rehabilitation* 1999;21:1-14.

54. Thompson C, Briggs M. Support for carers of people with Alzheimer's type dementia. *Cochrane Database of Systematic Reviews. Issue 3.* Oxford: Update Software, 2000.

55. Johnson WB, Lall R, Bongar B, Nordlund MD. The role of objective personality inventories in suicide risk assessment: An evaluation and proposal. *Suicide-and-Life-Threatening-Behavior* 1999;29:165-185.

56. Hawton K, Townsend E, Arensman E, et al. Psychosocial versus pharmacological treatments for deliberate self-harm (Cochrane Review). *In: The Cochrane Library, Issue 3, 2000* Oxford: Update Software, 2000.

57. Repper J. A review of the literature on the prevention of suicide through interventions in accident and emergency departments. *Journal of Clinical Nursing* 1999;8:3-12.

58. Van der Sande R, Buskens E, Allart E, Van der Graaf Y, Van Engeland H. Psychosocial intervention following suicide attempt: A systematic review of treatment interventions. *Acta-Psychiatrica-Scandinavica* 1997;96:43-50.

59. NHS CRD. Deliberate self-harm. *Effective Health Care* York: University of York, 1998.

60. NHS CRD. Mental health promotion in high risk groups. *Effective Health Care* York: University of York. 1997.

61. Badger, D., Nursten, J., Williams, P. and Woodward, M. Systematic review of the international literature on the epidemiology of mentally disordered offenders. *NHS CRD report 15,* York: University of York, 1999

62. Gilbody S, Pettigrew M. Rational decision-making in mental health: the role of systematic reviews. *The Journal of Mental Health Policy and Economics* 1999;2:99-106.

63. Beecham J, Knapp M, McGilloway S, et al. Leaving hospital ii: the cost-effectiveness of community care for former long-stay psychiatric hospital patients. *Journal of Mental Health* 1996;5:379-94.

64. Chiverton P, Tortoretti D, LaForest M, Walker PH. Bridging the gap between psychiatric hospitalization and community care: cost and quality outcomes. *Journal of the American Psychiatric Nurses Association* 1999;5:46-53.

65. Clark RE, Teague GB, Ricketts SK, et al. Cost-effectiveness of assertive community treatment versus standard case management for persons with co-occurring severe mental illness and substance use disorders. *Health Services Research* 1998;33:1285-1308.

66. Creed F, Mbaya P, Lancashire S, et al. Cost effectiveness of day and inpatient psychiatric treatment: results of a randomised controlled trial. *British Medical Journal* 1997:1381-5.

67. Dickey B, Fisher W, Siegel C, Altaffer F, Azeni H. The cost and outcomes of community-based care for the seriously mentally ill. *Health Services Research* 1997;32:599-614.

68. Drummond M, Mohide E, Tew M, et al. Economic evaluation of a support program for caregivers of demented elderly. *International Journal of Technology Assessment in Health Care* 1991;7:209-219.

69. Fontana A, Rosenheck R. Effectiveness and cost of the inpatient treatment of posttraumatic stress disorder - comparison of three models of treatment. *American Journal of Psychiatry* 1997:758-765.

70. French MT, Sacks S, de Leon G, Staines G, McKendrick K. Modified therapeutic community for mentally ill chemical abusers: outcomes and costs. (published erratum appears in Eval Health Prof 1999 Sep;22(3):399). *Evaluation & the Health Professions* 1999:60-85.

71. Gater R, Goldberg D, Jackson G, et al. The care of patients with chronic schizophrenia - a comparison between two services. *Psychological Medicine* 1997;27:1325-1336.

72. Goldberg D, Jackson G, Gater R, Campbell M, Jennett N. The treatment of common mental disorders by a community team based in primary care - a cost-effectiveness study. *Psychological Medicine* 1996;26:487-492.

73. Gournay K, Brooking J. The community psychiatric nurse in primary care: an economic analysis. *Journal of Advanced Nursing* 1995;22:769-778.

74. Group U. Cost-effectiveness of intensive v. standard case management for severe psychotic illness. *British Journal of Psychiatry* 2000;176:537-543.

75. Hawthorne WB, Green EE, Lohr JB, Hough R, Smith PG. Comparison of outcomes of acute care in short-term residential treatment and psychiatric hospital settings. *Psychiatric Services* 1999;50:401-406.

76. Hyde C, Bridges K, Goldberg D, et al. The evaultion of a hostel ward: a controlled study using modified cost-benefit analysis. *British Journal of Psychiatry* 1987;151:805-812.

77. Johnston S, Salkeld G, Sanderson K, et al. Intensive case management: a cost-effectiveness analysis. *Australian and New Zealand Journal of Psychiatry* 1998;32:551-559.

78. Lehman A, Dixon L, Hoch J, et al. Cost-effectiveness of assertive community treatment for homeless persons with severe mental illness. *British Journal of Psychiatry* 1999;174:346-352.

79. Mangen S, Paykel E, Griffith J, Burchell A, Mancini P. Cost-effectiveness of community psychiatric nurse or out-patient psychiatrist care of neurotic patients. *Psychological Medicine* 1983;13:407-416.

80. McCrone P, Beecham J, Knapp M. Community psychiatric nurse teams: cost-effectiveness of intensive support versus generic care. *British Journal of Psychiatry* 1994;164:218-221.

81. Merson S, Tyrer P, Carlen D, Johnson T. The cost of treatment of psychiatric emergencies - a comparison of hospital and community services. *Psychological Medicine* 1996;26:727-734.

82. Morriss R, Gask L, Ronalds C, et al. Cost-effectiveness of a new treatment for somatized mental disorder taught to GPs. *Family Practice* 1998;15:119-125.

83. Smith G, Rost K, Kashner T. A trial of the effect of a standardized psychiatric consultation on health outcomes and costs in somatizing patients. *Archives of General Psychiatry* 1995;52:238-243.

84. Tyrer P, Evans K, Gandhi N, et al. Randomised controlled trial of two models of care for discharged psychiatric patients. *British Medical Journal* 1998;316:106-109.

85. van Minnen A, Hoogduin C, Broekman T. Hospital vs. outreach treatment of patients with mental retardation and psychiatric disorders - a controlled study. *Acta Psychiatrica Scandinavica* 1997;95:515-522.

86. Von Korff M, Katon W, Bush T, et al. Treatment costs, cost offset, and cost-effectiveness of collaborative management of depression. *Psychosomatic Medicine* 1998;60:143-149.

87. Weisbrod B, Test M, Stein L. Alternative to mental hospital treatment: II Economic benefit-cost analysis. *Archives of General Psychiatry* 1980;37:400-405.

88. Wiersma D, Kluiter H, Nienhuis F, Ruphan M, R. G. Costs and benefits of hospital and day treatment with community care of affective and schizophrenic disorders. *British Journal of Psychiatry.* 1995;166:52-59,.

89. Wolff N, Helminiak T, Morse G, et al. Cost-effectiveness evaluation of three approaches to case management for homeless mentally ill clients. *American Journal of Psychiatry* 1997;153:341-348.

90. North Tyneside Community Health Council. Someone to talk to...Somewhere to go.Something to do. Exploring Options for the Development of 'Out-of-Hours' Mental Health Services., 1998

91. MIND. The MIND Model of a 24hr Crisis Service. 1995.

92. Appleby L, Shaw J, Amos T, et al. *Safer Services. Report of the National Confidential Inquiry into Suicide and Homicide by People with Mental Illness.* London: Department of Health 1999.

APPENDIX 1. SEARCH STRATEGY FOR IDENTIFYING SYSTEMATIC REVIEWS OF MENTAL HEALTH SERVICE DELIVERY INTERVENTIONS

Searches were undertaken to identify systematic reviews using the Cochrane Library and the administrative version of DARE (the Database of Abstracts of Reviews of Effectiveness).

A1.1 Cochrane Reviews
By using the search terms "mental or psych*" to retrieve reviews from CCTR

A1.2 DARE
The rationale for using the administrative version of DARE was that:
1) The database includes all systematic reviews identified by the NHS CRD team for potential inclusion in the public version of DARE.
2) It provides coverage of the following databases: Current Contents (1994 to date); MEDLINE (1994 to date); CINAHL (1994 to date); AMED (1994 to 1998); ERIC (1995 to 1998); PsycLIT (1995 to 1998); BIOSIS (1996 to 1998). These reviews are identified by using a pre-defined search strategy adapted for each of the databases.
3) It includes reviews identified by handsearching and reviews, which are not published.
4) It also includes reviews that have not yet been added to the public version of the database.

A1.3 PsycLIT
PsycLIT (on Silverplatter) were searched for the year 1999 using the strategy below. This will provide additional coverage of this database not achieved by using DARE.

#1	metaanaly*
#2	meta-analy* in ti
#3	meta-analy* in de
#4	cochrane* in ti
#5	(review* or overview*) in ti
#6	(review near literature) in ti
#7	(synthes* near (literature* or research or studies or data)) in ti
#8	(pooled near analys*) in ti
#9	((data near pool*) and studies) in ti
#10	(medline or medlars or pubmed or embase or cinahl or scisearch or psycinfo* or pyschinfo* or psyclit* or psychlit*) in ti
#11	(medline or medlars or pubmed or embase or cinahl or scisearch or psycinfo* or pyschinfo* or psyclit* or psychlit*) in de
#12	((hand or manual* or database* or computer*) near search*) in ti
#13	((hand or manual* or database* or computer*) near search*) in de
#14	((electronic or bibliograpohic*) near (database* or (data near base*))) in ti
#15	((electronic or bibliograpohic*) near (database* or (data near base*))) in ab
#16	(review* or overview*) in ti
#17	(systematic* or methodologic* or quantitative* or research* or literature or studies or trial* or effective*) in ti
#18	#16 near #17
#19	#1 or #2 or #3 or #4 or #5 or #6 or #7 or #8 or #9 or #10 or #11 or #12 or #13 or #14 or #15 or #18
#20	retrospective* near review*
#21	case* near review*
#22	record* near review*
#23	patient* near review*
#24	patient* near chart*
#25	peer near review*
#26	(chart* near review*) in ti
#27	(chart* near review*) in ab
#28	(case* near report*) in ti
#29	(case* near report*) in ab
#30	(case control* stud*) in ti

#31	(case control* stud*) in ab
#32	(prospective stud*) in ti
#33	(prospective stud*) in ab
#34	(rat or rats or mouse or mice or hamster or hamsters or animal or animals or dog or dogs or cat or cats or bovine or sheep) in ti
#35	(rat or rats or mouse or mice or hamster or hamsters or animal or animals or dog or dogs or cat or cats or bovine or sheep) in ab
#36	(rat or rats or mouse or mice or hamster or hamsters or animal or animals or dog or dogs or cat or cats or bovine or sheep) in de
#37	#20 or #21 or #22 or #23 or #24 or #25 or #26 or #27 or #28 or #29 or #30 or #31 or #32 or #33 or #34 or #35 or #36
#38	#19 not #37
#39	animal
#40	human
#41	#39 not (#39 and #40)
#42	#38 not #41
#43	amino acid sequence
#44	base sequence
#45	chromosome mapping
#46	molecular sequence data
#47	gene library
#48	dna complementary
#49	ribosomal proteins
#50	clone cells
#51	mutation
#52	protein binding
#53	gene expression regulation
#54	#43 or #44 or #45 or #46 or #47 or #48 or #49 or #50 or #51 or #52 or #53
#55	#42 not #54
#57	#55 and (PY >= "1999")

A1.4 EMBASE

EMBASE (on Silverplatter) were searched for the period 1994-Dec 1999 using the strategy below:

The searches below are from: A:\EMBMENT.HIS.

#1	explode "mental-health-service"/ all subheadings
#2	explode "mental-health-care"/ all subheadings
#3	explode "mental-health-center"/ all subheadings
#4	explode "mental-health"/ all subheadings
#5	explode "community-mental-health"/ all subheadings
#6	explode "community-mental-health-center"/ all subheadings
#7	explode "mental-hospital"/ all subheadings
#8	explode "psychiatric-department"/ all subheadings
#9	explode "psychosocial-care"/ all subheadings
#10	explode "liaison-psychiatry"/ all subheadings
#11	explode "crisis-intervention"/ all subheadings
#12	explode "suicide"/ all subheadings
#13	explode "suicide-attempt"/ all subheadings
#14	mental or psychiatr*
#15	explode "health-education"/ all subheadings
#16	#14 and #15
#17	explode "health-promotion"/ all subheadings
#18	#14 and #17
#19	explode "emergency-health-service"/ all subheadings
#20	#14 and #19
#21	explode "caregiver"/ all subheadings
#22	#14 and #21
#23	acute psychiatric car*
#24	acute emergency car*
#25	acute respite

#26	acute asylum
#27	assertive outreach
#28	assertive community outreach
#29	assertive community treatment
#30	asylum care
#31	case management
#32	care management and #14
#33	care program* approach*
#34	community mental health service*
#35	community mental hygiene service*
#36	community mental health center*
#37	community mental health centre*
#38	community treatment unit*
#39	community mental health team*
#40	crisis intervention service*
#41	crisis service*
#42	crisis care
#43	mental health services
#44	mental health clinic*
#45	mental health unit*
#46	mental institute*
#47	mental institution*
#48	mental health centre*
#49	mental health assess*
#50	mental health liaison service*
#51	mental care
#52	mental help
#53	mental service*
#54	mental ward*
#55	mental health crisis
#56	mental health crises
#57	psychiatric care
#58	psychiatric centr*
#59	psychiatric clinic*
#60	psychiatric hospital*
#61	psychiatric unit*
#62	psychiatric ward*
#63	psychiatric emergency
#64	psychiatric urgen*
#65	community psychiatr*
#66	emergency psychiatr*
#67	total psychiatr* service*
#68	home treatment* and (mental or psychiatr*)
#69	suicide prevention
#70	respite care and (mental or psychiatr*)
#71	safe house* and (mental or psychiatr*)
#72	sanctuary and (mental or psychiatr*)
#73	outreach service and (mental or psychiatr*)
#74	brief hospitali?ation and (mental or psychiatr*)
#75	psychotic relapse
#76	short term care and (mental or psychiatr*)
#77	daily living program* and (mental or psychiatr*)
#78	home care and (mental or psychiatr*)
#79	home based care and (mental or psychiatr*)
#80	community oriented treat* and (mental or psychiatr*)
#81	community orientated treat* and (mental or psychiatr*)
#82	(carer* or relative* or family or families) near3 support*
#83	#82 and (mental or psychiatr*)
#84	helpline* and (mental or psychiatr*)
#85	hotline* and (mental or psychiatr*)

#86 telephone* and (mental or psychiatr*)
#87 #84 or #85 or #86
#88 #1 or #2 or #3 or #4 or #5 or #6 or #7 or #8 or #9 or #10 or #11 or #12 or #13
#89 #16 or #18 or #20 or #22 or #23 or #24 or #25 or #26 or #27 or #28 or #29 or #30 or #31 or #32 or #33 or #34 or #35 or #36 or #37 or #38 or #39 or #40
#90 #41 or #42 or #43 or #44 or #45 or #46 or #47 or #48 or #49 or #50 or #51 or #52 or #53 or #54 or #55 or #56 or #57 or #58 or #59 or #60
#91 #61 or #62 or #63 or #64 or #65 or #66 or #67 or #68 or #69 or #70 or #71 or #72 or #73 or #74 or #75 or #76 or #77 or #78 or #80 or #81 or #83 or #87
#92 #88 or #89 or #90 or #91
#93 "meta-analysis"/ all subheadings
#94 metaanalys* in ti,ab
#95 meta-analys* in ti, ab
#96 meta analys* in ti, ab
#97 cochrane in ti,ab,de
#98 (review* or overview*) in ti
#99 review in dt
#100 synthes* near3 ((literature* or research* or studies or data) in ti,ab)
#101 (pooled analys*) in ti,ab
#102 (data near2 pool*) and studies
#103 (medline or medlars or embase or cinahl or scisearch or psychinfo or psycinfo or psychlit or psyclit) in ti,ab
#104 ((hand or manual or database* or computer*) near2 search*) in ti,ab
#105 ((electronic or bibliographic*) near2 (database* or data base*)) in ti,ab
#106 (review* or overview*) near10 ((systematic* or methodologic* or quantitativ* or research* or literature* or studies or trial* or effective*) in ab)
#107 #93 or #94 or #95 or #96 or #97 or #98 or #99 or #100 or #101 or #102 or #103 or #104 or #105 or #106
#108 (retrospective* near2 review*) in ti,ab,de
#109 (case* near2 review*)in ti,ab,de
#110 (record* near2 review*) in ti,ab,de
#111 (patient* near2 review*)in ti,ab,de
#112 (patient* near2 chart*)in ti,ab,de
#113 (peer near2 review*) in ti,ab,de
#114 (chart* ncar2 review*) in ti,ab,de
#115 (case* near2 report*) in ti,ab,de
#116 (rat or rats or mouse or mice or hamster or hamsters or animal or animals or dog or dogs or cat or cats or bovine or sheep) in ti,ab,de
#117 #108 or #109 or #110 or #111 or #112 or #113 or #114 or #115 or #116
#118 #117 not (#117 and #107)
#119 #107 not #118
#120 editorial in dt
#121 letter in dt
#122 #120 or #121
#123 #119 not #122
#124 explode "animal"/ all subheadings
#125 explode "human"/ all subheadings
#126 #124 not (#124 and #125)
#127 explode "nonhuman"/ all subheadings
#128 explode "human"/ all subheadings
#129 #127 not (#127 and #128)
#130 #126 or #129
#131 #123 not #130
#132 #92 and #131

A1.5 The Internet

The Internet was searched for relevant systematic reviews. Particular emphasis was put on searching the web sites of organisations indexed in 'Netting the Evidence. A ScHARR Introduction to Evidence Based Practice on the Internet' (http://www.shef.ac.uk/~scharr/ir/netting.html)

A1.6 Additional searching.
The Advisory Board suggested some additional search terms and further searches were carried out as below.

A1.6.1 Additional searching of MEDLINE (on Silverplatter) (1966-2000/06) was carried out using the strategy below combined with a systematic reviews search strategy. This retrieved 121 additional records.

#1	explode "Mental-Disorders"/ all subheadings
#2	(mental or psychiatr*) in ti,ab,mesh
#3	#1 or #2
#4	explode "Self-Injurious-Behavior"/ all subheadings
#5	self-harm
#6	parasuicide
#7	explode "Suicide"/ all subheadings
#8	explode "Emergency-Medical-Services"/ all subheadings
#9	explode "Emergency-Service-Hospital"/ all subheadings
#10	accident near emergency
#11	explode "Referral-and-Consultation"/ all subheadings
#12	explode "Ambulatory-Care"/ all subheadings
#13	explode "Outpatient-Clinics-Hospital"/ all subheadings
#14	explode "Commitment-of-Mentally-Ill"/ all subheadings
#15	outpatient* service*
#16	outpatient* unit*
#17	outpatient* clinic*
#18	explode "Risk-Assessment"/ all subheadings
#19	"Bed-Occupancy"/ all subheadings
#20	explode "Length-of-Stay"/ all subheadings
#21	explode "Patient-Admission"/ all subheadings
#22	"Patient-Readmission"/ all subheadings
#23	short hospitali?ation
#24	revolv* door*
#25	primary care
#26	general practice
#27	general practitioner*
#28	"Family-Practice"/ all subheadings
#29	"Physicians-Family"/ all subheadings
#30	secure accommodation
#31	explode "Prisons"/ all subheadings
#32	key worker*
#33	care plan*
#34	survivor*
#35	explode "Self-Help-Groups"/ all subheadings
#36	explode "Patient-Advocacy"/ all subheadings
#37	approved social work*
#38	"Employment-Supported"/ all subheadings
#39	clubhouse
#40	employment train*
#41	support* employment
#42	#3 or #4 or #5 or #6 or #7
#43	#8 or #9 or #10 or #11 or #12 or #13 or #14 or #15 or #16 or #17 or #18 or #19 or #20
#44	#21 or #22 or #23 or #24 or #25 or #26 or #27 or #28 or #29 or #30 or #31 or #32 or #33 or #34 or #35 or #36 or #37 or #38 or #39 or #40 or #41
#45	#43 or #44
#46	#45 and #42

A1.6.2 Additional searching of EMBASE (on Silverplatter) (1994-2000/05) was carried out using the strategy below combined with a systematic reviews search strategy. This retrieved 2837 additional records.

#	Search
#1	explode "mental-disease"/ all subheadings
#2	(mental or psychiatr*) in ti,ab,de
#3	#1 or #2
#4	"automutilation"/ all subheadings
#5	self-harm
#6	parasuicide
#7	"suicide"/ all subheadings
#8	"suicide-attempt"/ all subheadings
#9	"emergency-health-service"/ all subheadings
#10	accident near emergency
#11	"patient-referral"/ all subheadings
#12	"ambulatory-care"/ all subheadings
#13	"outpatient-department"/ all subheadings
#14	"forensic-psychiatry"/ all subheadings
#15	outpatient* service*
#16	outpatient* unit*
#17	outpatient* clinic*
#18	"risk-assessment"/ all subheadings
#19	"hospital-bed-utilization"/ all subheadings
#20	bed occupancy
#21	"length-of-stay"/ all subheadings
#22	"hospital-admission"/ all subheadings
#23	patient admission
#24	short hospitali?ation
#25	revolv* door*
#26	"primary-medical-care"/ all subheadings
#27	primary care
#28	general practice
#29	general practitioner*
#30	family practice
#31	family practitioner*
#32	secure accommodation
#33	"prison"/ all subheadings
#34	key worker*
#35	care plan*
#36	survivor*
#37	"self-help"/ all subheadings
#38	"human-rights"/ all subheadings
#39	advocacy
#40	approved social work*
#41	"employment"/ all subheadings
#42	supported employment
#43	employment train*
#44	clubhouse*
#45	#3 or #4 or #5 or #6 or #7 or #8
#46	#9 or #10 or #11 or #12 or #13 or #14 or #15 or #16 or #17 or #18 or #19 or #20
#47	#21 or #22 or #23 or #24 or #25 or #26 or #27 or #28 or #29 or #30
#48	#31 or #32 or #33 or #34 or #35 or #36 or #37 or #38 or #39 or #40 or #41 or #42 or #43 or #44
#49	#46 or #47 or #48
#50	#45 and #49

APPENDIX 2. CRITERIA FOR ASSESSING QUALITY OF REVIEWS OF EFFECTIVENESS (DARE INCLUSION CRITERIA)

1. Does the review answer a well defined question?

A good review should focus on a well defined question, making the objectives of the review easy to understand. The most important components in a review question include the target population, health care intervention and outcomes of interest.

2. Was a substantial effort made to search for all the relevant literature?

It should be stated in the review which databases were searched, what time period was covered, and which search terms were used. In addition, details of handsearching and efforts to identify unpublished studies should be reported.

3. Are the inclusion/exclusion criteria reported and are they appropriate?

Criteria for the inclusion of individual studies in a review have two major dimensions: relevance and validity. A relevant study should be useful to answer review questions in terms of patients, intervention and outcomes. The validity issue is related to the methodological standard of an individual study.

4. Is the validity of included studies adequately assessed?

The validity or quality criteria which were assessed (such as blinding of assessment, concealment of randomisation, adjustment for case-mix) are considered here.

5. Is sufficient detail of the individual studies presented?

Details of the individual studies included in the review include study design, sample size in each study group, patient characteristics, description of interventions, settings, outcome measures, follow-up, drop out rate, effectiveness results and side-effects. The importance of study details may differ for different review topics.

6. Have the primary studies been combined or summarised appropriately?

Consideration is given to whether the studies were combined using a statistical method (Mantel-Haenszel, Peto, fixed effects, random effects etc) and which factors were taken into account when weighting the studies listed (sample size, quality score etc). In a narrative synthesis the method of study selection and weighting will be considered.

Studies had to meet at least four of these criteria in order to be included in the review.

APPENDIX 3. DATA EXTRACTION TABLES FOR SYSTEMATIC REVIEWS OF HEALTH SERVICE DELIVERY INTERVENTIONS
NSF standard 1. Mental Health Promotion

Review	Review Methodology	Included trial details	Participants	Intervention details	Outcomes	Results	Author's conclusions
Author Tilford et al[10] **Date published (date last updated)*** 1997 **Title** Effectiveness of mental health promotion interventions: a review **Review type** non-Cochrane **Objectives** To prepare a systematic review of evidence of the effectiveness of interventions aiming to promote health and/or prevent mental disorder	**Search strategy** MEDLINE, PsycLIT, CINAHL, ASSIA, and Eric were searched for relevant trials. Relevant journals, indexes and abstracts were handsearched. The searches were restricted to English language articles and to the years 1980-1995. **Quality assessment** Not stated, but methodological quality of the included studies was discussed **Statistical analysis** Narrative summary **Quality score (assessed by reviewers):** 5	**Types of studies** RCTs, quasi-RCTs, and uncontrolled studies **Number of studies included** Forty papers were included for the adult group (19 RCTs, 21 before and after studies) with a total of 7,332 participants **Years of studies:** 1980-1995 **Countries where studies undertaken** UK: 9 USA and Canada: 18 Norway and Sweden: 3 Australasia: 2 Unknown: 8	General population, and people at risk of mental illness. The authors excluded studies of: psychiatric in-patients, patients in secondary treatment setting or major psychiatric disorders, workplace setting, alcohol misuse and drug treatments.	Any activity undertaken with the goal of improving mental health or modifying its determinants or preventing mental illness or risk factors associated with it. Interventions were carried out as part of a specialist health promotion practice or the practice of other professionals (not necessarily labelled as health promotion) and within health-care, educational and community settings. Interventions included mass media, general lifestyle interventions, prevention of marital distress and interventions for at-risk adults (e.g. parents, women at risk of, or experiencing depression, ethnic minorities, people with suicidal intentions) and carers.	Promotion of positive mental health; prevention of specified mental disorders and outcomes; development of the major intermediate factors associated with mental health/prevention of mental disorder	Mass media interventions provide evidence of the limited but valuable contribution that can be made to modifying knowledge and attitudes to mental illness. General health promotion programmes can have an impact on a range of outcomes. There was some evidence for the effectiveness of brief interventions at the time of critical illness. Studies on first-time parent indicate the difficulties of achieving defined goals. There is evidence that 'listening visits' and other counselling interventions may be important for the early detection and reduction of postnatal depression. .	Mental health objectives should be addressed in the context of general health promotion interventions. More consideration should be given to the role of the mass media, and brief interventions for coping with critical illness within a family, and interventions for coping with longer term life changes. More work is needed on interventions aimed at preventing depression. There should be more community-based structured group schemes for women who feel depressed but who have not yet been professionally diagnosed. 'Listening visits' should be introduced, to help prevent and treat postnatal depression.

*Cochrane reviews only

NSF standards two and three: primary care & access to services

Review	Review Methodology	Included trial details	Participants	Intervention details	Outcomes	Results	Author's conclusions
Author Abi-Aad et al[17] **Date published (date last updated)*** 2000 (expected end 2001) **Title** Primary and community health care professionals in hospital emergency departments: effects on process and outcome of care and resources **Review type** Cochrane protocol **Objectives** To investigate the effects of locating primary and community professionals to manage patients with minor injury or illness in the hospital emergency department	**Search strategy** The specialised register of EPOC, Cochrane Controlled Trials Register, MEDLINE (1966-2000), EMBASE (1981-2000); HealthStar (1975-2000), Cinahl (1980-2000); PsycLIT (1974-), Sociological Abstracts, ASSIA, Social Science and Science Citation Indexes (1981-2000), HMIC Databases, SIGLE (all available years), UK Economic and Social Research Council Register of Funded Research and UK National Centre for Primary Care Research and Development database will be searched for trials **Quality assessment** Data on validity will be extracted using the EPOC data extraction checklist **Statistical analysis** Results will be reported in natural units and post-intervention mean differences will be reported or calculated where possible. If trials are located which use similar comparisons and units, their results may be combined. **Quality score (assessed by reviewers):** N/a	**Types of studies** RCTs, controlled before and after studies (CBA), and interrupted time series studies (ITS) **Number of studies included** N/a **Years of studies:** N/a **Countries where studies undertaken** N/a	Patients with minor illness or injury attending hospital emergency departments. Primary health and community care professionals include any staff member with a recognised primary or community care specialism. Examples include: general practitioners, nurses with primary or community care qualifications (for example nurse practitioners, mental health workers (for example community psychiatric nurse).	Interventions in which primary or community care professionals provide care for new attenders at the hospital emergency department	Proportion of patients receiving: diagnostic interventions; treatments; referral to specialist care; hospital admission; referral to outpatient or follow-up clinic. Proportion of patients discharged with advice for self management. Objective measures of repeat attendances to emergency departments. Objective measures of subsequent utilisation of primary care services. Objective measures of general health status or functioning. Also staff and prescription costs.	N/a	N/a

*Cochrane reviews only

Review	Review Methodology	Included trial details	Participants	Intervention details	Outcomes	Results	Author's conclusions
Author Bower and Sibbald [15,16] **Date published (date last updated)*** 2000 **Title** On-site mental health workers in primary care: effects on professional practice **Review type** Cochrane review and published review (results taken from Cochrane review) **Objectives** To assess the effects of on-site MHWs in primary care on the clinical behaviour of primary care providers (PCPs).	**Search strategy** MEDLINE (1966-1998), PsycINFO (1984-1998), EMBASE (1980-1998), the Cochrane Clinical Trials Register, the specialised register of the Effective Practice and Organisation of Care (EPOC) Group, and Counselling in Primary Care Trust.Lit database were searched for relevant trials. The reference lists of all identified studies were also searched. **Quality assessment** The quality of all eligible trials was assessed using the criteria described by the EPOC group **Statistical analysis** Narrative summary **Quality score (assessed by reviewers): 7**	**Types of studies** RCTs, controlled clinical trials (CCTs), controlled before and after studies (CBAs) and interrupted time series (ITSs) **Number of studies included** 38 studies involving more than 460 PCPs and more than 3880 patients. **Years of studies:** 1982-1998 **Countries where studies undertaken** UK: 29 USA: 6 Australasia: 2 Germany: 1	Primary care providers (PCPs). In order to ensure comparability of interventions, the review is restricted to PCPs who fulfil the following definition: 'PCPs are medical health professionals providing first contact and on-going care to patients, regardless of the patient's age, gender or presenting problem.'	The main requirements for interventions to be included in the review were: (1) services provided by an on-site MHW represent a separate and distinct activity and are not solely part of normal primary care consultations. (2) the MHW is employed by or attached to the PCP organisation and works 'on-site' i.e. the PCP and MHW work for at least part of the time in geographical proximity as part of the same clinical team. The comparison group was PCP organisations without employed or attached MHWs.	1. PCP detection rates and diagnostic accuracy. 2. PCP off-site mental health referral behaviour. 3. PCP prescribing behaviour. Any other relevant and reliable PCP outcome measures that were reported (e.g. increases in consultation length, number of patient contacts, types of services offered).	There was some evidence that 'replacement' model MHWs achieved significant short-term reductions in PCP psychotropic prescribing and mental health referral, but the effects were not reliable. Consultation rates were also reduced, but with even less evidence of a consistent effect. There were no indirect effects in prescribing behaviour on the wider population and no consistent pattern to the impact on referrals. There was some evidence that 'consultation-liaison' model MHWs had a direct effect on PCP prescribing behaviour when used as part of complex, multifaceted interventions.	This review does not support the hypothesis that adding MHWs to primary care provider organisations in 'replacement' models causes a significant or enduring change in PCP behaviour. 'Consultation-liaison' interventions may cause changes in psychotropic prescribing, but these seem short-term and limited to patients under the direct care of the MHW. Longer-term studies are needed to assess the degree to which demonstrated effects endure over time.

*Cochrane reviews only

Review	Author	Review Methodology	Included trial details	Participants	Intervention details	Outcomes	Results	Author's conclusions
Author Boyle et al [20] **Date published (date last updated)*** 1999 (expected mid-2000) **Title** Interventions available for the treatment of anorexia nervosa specialist clinics versus non-specialist clinics **Review type** Cochrane protocol **Objectives** To perform a systematic review of all RCTs dealing with interventions for anorexia nervosa (DSM III / IV) and meta-analysis if appropriate		**Search strategy** MEDLINE, LILACS, prospectively) PsycLIT, Psyndex, SIGLE, MRC database, EMBASE, and conference abstracts will be searched for relevant trials. Reference lists will also be searched and contact is being maintained with pharmaceutical companies to gain access to trials. **Quality assessment** Each study will be assessed and described for the strength of its internal validity and statistical power **Statistical analysis** If a meta-analysis is appropriate on the basis of the studies available, the data will be analysed using Review Manager software which will facilitate the calculation of CIs and odds ratios (OR) **Quality score (assessed by reviewers):** N/a	**Types of studies** RCTs which measured and reported on clinically relevant outcomes including at least one year of follow-up measurement **Number of studies included** N/a **Years of studies:** N/a **Countries where studies undertaken** N/a	Adults aged between 15-25 at the time of admission to the trial and present with identifiable criteria consistent with DSM III / IV for anorexia nervosa	The trials will include treatment elements which could be expected to be available in in-patient or residential settings. Both psychological and pharmaceutical treatments will be considered, as will those which look at the setting in which treatment happens (eg, whether inpatient, outpatient, day care or specialist centre).	A range of outcome measures is available for assessing the effectiveness of treatment for anorexia nervosa with different combinations of physical, psychological and social elements. The focus of the study will be those outcome measures such as the Morgan Russell scale which will consider all these factors in addition to Body Mass Index alone.	N/a	N/a

*Cochrane reviews only

Review	Author	Review Methodology	Included trial details	Participants	Intervention details	Outcomes	Results	Author's conclusions
Author Grimshaw et al[18] **Date published (date last updated)*** 1999 (expected end 2000) **Title** Interventions to improve physician referrals from primary to secondary care **Review type** Cochrane protocol **Objectives** To identify which interventions have been evaluated to change or improve referral from primary care to secondary care. To estimate the effectiveness of interventions to change or improve referral from primary care to secondary care		**Search strategy** MEDLINE (1966 - 1998), EMBASE (1980 - 1998), PsycLIT (1887 - 1998), CINAHL (1982 - 1998), HealthStar (1975 - 1998) The Primary - Secondary Care database, The Cochrane Library - Issue 2, 1999, and the EPOC specialised register will be searched for relevant trials. In addition several journals will be handsearched, and an international group of experts (who have published papers on hospital referrals) will be contacted to identify further studies. **Quality assessment** The review will be conducted by using methods described by EPOC **Statistical analysis** Given the expected substantial heterogeneity of interventions and methods across studies, it is not anticipated that it will be sensible to use meta-analysis to pool the results of studies. Instead the results of will presented in tabular form and a narrative summary given. **Quality score (assessed by reviewers):** N/a	**Types of studies** RCTs, controlled clinical trials (CCTs), controlled before and after studies (CBAs) and interrupted time series (ITSs) **Number of studies included** N/a **Years of studies:** N/a **Countries where studies undertaken** N/a	Primary care physicians, defined broadly as any medically qualified physician who provides primary health care. Primary care physicians include general practitioners, family doctors, family physicians, family practitioners and other physicians working in primary health care settings who fulfil primary health care tasks. Secondary care physicians working in hospitals (clinic, outpatient clinic and emergency department) or community settings.	Interventions to change or improve referrals from primary care physicians to secondary care (including outpatient, accident and emergency and inpatient referrals). To be included, studies have to report explicitly that influencing referral was a primary objective of the intervention to be included.	Objective measures of provider performance in a health care setting (for example referral rates or appropriateness of referral) or health outcomes will be included	N/a	N/a

*Cochrane reviews only

Review	Review Methodology	Included trial details	Participants	Intervention details	Outcomes	Results	Author's conclusions
Author Haynes et al[21] **Date published (date last updated)*** 1999 **Title** Interventions for helping patients to follow prescriptions for medications **Review type** Cochrane review **Objectives** To update an ongoing review summarising the results of randomised controlled trials (RCTs) of interventions to help patients follow prescriptions for medications, focusing on trials that measured both adherence and clinical outcomes	**Search strategy** MEDLINE, CINAHL, The Cochrane Library, International Pharmaceutical Abstracts (IPA), PsychInfo, Sociofile, and HSTAR were searched to July 1998. Bibliographies in articles on patient adherence, articles in the reviewers' personal collections were also searched and contact was made with authors. **Quality assessment** Not stated **Statistical analysis** Narrative summary and data reported in tables **Quality score (assessed by reviewers):** 5	**Types of studies** RCTs with at least 80% follow-up of each group studied and, for long-term treatments, at least six months follow-up for studies with positive initial findings **Number of studies included** 19 RCTs (total number of participants not stated) **Years of studies:** 1972-1998 **Countries where studies undertaken** Not stated	People who were prescribed medication for a medical disorder (including psychiatric disorders)	Interventions of any sort intended to affect adherence with prescribed, self-administered medications	Measures of both medication adherence and treatment outcome. For long-term regimens, studies with initially positive findings were required to have at least 6 months follow-up from the time of patient entry.	For short-term treatments, one study, of counselling and written information, showed an effect on adherence and clinical outcome. 10/19 interventions for long-term treatments reported in 17 RCTs were associated with improvements in adherence, but only nine interventions led to improvements in treatment outcomes. Almost all of the interventions that were effective for long-term care were complex. Even the most effective interventions did not lead to large improvements in adherence and treatment outcomes. Two studies showed that telling patients about adverse effects of treatment did not affect their adherence.	The full benefits of medications cannot be realised at currently achievable levels of adherence. Current methods of improving adherence for chronic health problems are mostly complex and not very effective. More studies of innovative approaches to assist patients to follow medication prescriptions are needed.

*Cochrane reviews only

Review	Review Methodology	Included trial details	Participants	Intervention details	Outcomes	Results	Author's conclusions
Author Hulscher et al [13] **Date published (date last updated)*** 1999 **Title** Interventions to improve the delivery of preventive services in primary care **Review type** Published and Cochrane protocol **Objectives** To determine the effectiveness of interventions aimed at primary care clinicians to improve the delivery of preventive services	**Search strategy** MEDLINE (1966-1995), the contents tables of 21 scientific journals (1980-1995) and the EPOC register of trials were searched for relevant trials **Quality assessment** Eligible studies were independently assessed by at least two reviewers using the EPOC data collection checklist which concerned methodological aspects (e.g. research design and sample size) **Statistical analysis** Narrative summary. Results from the trials were reported in tables **Quality score (assessed by reviewers):** 6	**Types of studies** RCTs or controlled before-after studies (CBA). Interrupted time-series analyses were only included when a control group or condition was used. **Number of studies included** 58 studies (only one was relevant to this scoping review - a RCT with 32 participants) **Years of studies:** Relevant study was undertaken in 1988 **Countries where studies undertaken** Not stated	Any primary care professional who is responsible for patient care. Professionals deliver primary care if they are directly accessible to patients for all types of health problems. General practitioners, family physicians, and practice nurse are all examples of primary care providers.	Any type of educational, organisational, financial or regulatory intervention aimed at improving primary prevention (activities aimed at preventing diseases) or secondary prevention (early detection of diseases), including counselling, vaccinations and screening; where the targeted preventive services entail some implicit or explicit recommended course of action. The majority of studies included in the review were not relevant to this scoping review. They included trials of screening procedures, immunisation and health related behaviours such as cigarette smoking.	Any objective measure of professional performance or patient health outcomes. Self-reported behaviour outcomes were included only if they concerned patient-specific outcomes. Attitude and knowledge outcomes were excluded.	The 58 studies included comprised 86 comparisons between intervention and control groups. Most interventions were found to be effective in some studies but not others. Only one study looked at the outcomes of mental health and few details are provided. The intervention was multifaceted and included physician reminders. The mean performance score before the intervention was 7.00 in the intervention group and 15.00 in the control group. After the intervention, the mean intervention score was 20.0 in the intervention group and 13.0 in the control group. The difference in post intervention score was not significant.	Effective interventions to increase preventive activities in primary care are available. Detailed studies are needed to identify factors that influence the effectiveness of different interventions.

*Cochrane reviews only

Review	Author	Review Methodology	Included trial details	Participants	Intervention details	Outcomes	Results	Author's conclusions
Author Kroenke et al[12] **Date published (date last updated)*** 2000 **Title** Interventions to improve provider diagnosis and treatment of mental disorders in primary care - A critical review of the literature **Review type** non-Cochrane **Objectives** To assess whether interventions aimed at providers can improve the diagnosis, treatment and clinical outcomes of depression and other mental disorders in primary care		**Search strategy** MEDLINE (1966-1998) was searched. Articles were also identified from bibliographies of review articles and retrieved articles **Quality assessment** Not stated, however the results were compared by study design (RCT/non-RCT) **Statistical analysis** Narrative summary. Studies were classified as positive for an outcome if the intervention resulted in a statistically significant result (p<0.005). Magnitude of a positive effect was also reported. **Quality score (assessed by reviewers):** 5	**Types of studies** RCTs, pre-post or non RCTs **Number of studies included** 48 studies (27 RCTs, and 21 non-RCTs) with a total of 27, 284 participants **Years of studies:** 1976-1998 **Countries where studies undertaken** USA: 33 UK: 10 Canada: 1 Australia: 1 India: 1 Sweden: 1 Saudi Arabia: 1	Providers of care in the primary setting	The primary focus of the intervention was on improving the recognition and/or management of one or more mental disorders in the primary care setting. Predisposing (e.g. reading materials, didactic training sessions), enabling (e.g., screening tools for physician use, mental health professional consultation), and reinforcing (e.g., supervised rotations, monitoring patient treatment) interventions were used in 34, 24, and 17 studies, respectively.	Provider knowledge, attitudes or skill, process of care (e.g. diagnostic rates or treatment actions); and clinical outcomes (e.g. symptom severity, functional status, health carte costs, satisfaction with care)	Improved diagnosis of health care providers was reported in 18 of 23 (78%) of the studies examining this outcome and improved treatment in 14 of 20 studies (70%). Clinical improvement in psychiatric symptoms or functional status was documented in 4 of 11 and 4 of 8 studies (36% and 50%, respectively). Considerable study heterogeneity precluded subjecting the literature synthesis to a formal meta-analysis, preventing any demonstration of an association between efficacy of an intervention and any specific variables.	A variety of interventions and further research may be effective in improving the recognition and management of health care providers in primary care.

*Cochrane reviews only

Review	Review Methodology	Included trial details	Participants	Intervention details	Outcomes	Results	Author's conclusions
Author Ray et al [19] **Date published (date last updated)*** Sept 1997 **Title** Caregiver support for postpartum depression **Review type** Cochrane review **Objectives** To assess the effect of professional and/or social support interventions for the treatment of postpartum depression	**Search strategy** The review has drawn on the register developed for the Pregnancy and Childbirth Group as a whole **Quality assessment** Details of randomisation, concealment allocation, blinding and exclusions from data analyses were recorded and evaluated. A rating was assigned to each trial, based on the quality categories described in the Cochrane Collaboration Handbook. Only trials in categories A or B were included in this review. **Statistical analysis** The OR and 95% confidence intervals were calculated for categorical results of comparable trials. Results were pooled using a fixed effect model. **Quality score (assessed by reviewers): 7**	**Types of studies** RCTs **Number of studies included** 2 RCTs with a total of 137 women **Years of studies:** 1989-1997 **Countries where studies undertaken** UK	All primiparous or multiparous women and their partners who had a live infant at the time they were admitted into a trial and were identified as depressed postnatally were included. Therefore, women experiencing second Trimester terminations were excluded. A broad definition of postpartum depression was used that excluded 'postpartum blues' and ignored the cause or timing of onset of the depression, to include women who were determined to be clinically depressed during the first six months postpartum.	All types of professional and/or social support including emotional support, counselling, tangible assistance and information delivered by telephone, home or clinic visits, or individual or group sessions, compared with any form of usual care for depressed mothers	All unbiased estimates of the effectiveness of professional and/or social support interventions for the treatment of postpartum depression on indicators of maternal and family morbidity, including the duration and resolution of the depression and other indicators of social functioning	The common outcome for both trials was depression at 25 weeks postpartum, which was significantly reduced in the groups receiving additional support (OR 0.34; 95% CI 0.17, 0.69).	There is some indication that professional and/or social support may help in the treatment of postpartum depression. The types of support should be investigated to assess which models are most effective. While there is good theoretical justification for the potential benefits of social support in the resolution of postpartum depression, it would be premature to make practice recommendations based upon two small trials. Only 111 women have been studied to date.

*Cochrane reviews only

Review	Review Methodology	Included trial details	Participants	Intervention details	Outcomes	Results	Author's conclusions
Author Schulberg et al[23] **Date published (date last updated)*** 1998 **Title** Treating major depression in primary care practice - an update of the agency for health care policy and research practice guidelines **Review type** non-Cochrane **Objectives** Not stated	**Search strategy** The Cochrane Collaboration Depression, Anxiety and Neurosis Controlled Trials Register was searched for trials published between 1992-1998 **Quality assessment** Not stated **Statistical analysis** Narrative summary **Quality score (assessed by reviewers): 4**	**Types of studies** RCTs which used an intention to treat analysis **Number of studies included** Not stated, but only two areas of the review were relevant to this scoping review **Years of studies:** Not stated **Countries where studies undertaken** Not stated	People with major depression treated in primary care	Interventions relevant to this scoping review were: weekly versus bi-weekly visits; transfer of antidepressant pharmacotherapy from specialist to primary care; transfer of depression-specific psychosocial therapies from specialist to primary care.	Effectiveness in treating depression	The evidence indicates that both antidepressants and time-limited depression-targeted psychotherapies are efficacious when transferred from psychiatric to primary care settings. No studies directly assessed the link between visit frequency and outcome. However, there is some evidence to suggest that more frequent visits during acute phase improve clinical outcome.	Studies to date suggest that improving treatment of depression in primary care requires properly organised treatment programmes, regular patient follow-up, monitoring of treatment adherence, and a prominent role for the mental health specialist as educator, consultant and clinician for the more severely ill. Future research should focus on how guidelines are best implemented in routine practice.

*Cochrane reviews only

NSF STANDARDS FOUR AND FIVE: EFFECTIVE SERVICES FOR PEOPLE WITH SEVERE MENTAL ILLNESS

Review	Review Methodology	Included trial details	Participants	Intervention details	Outcomes	Results	Author's conclusions
Author Almaraz-Serrano et al [48] **Date published (date last updated)*** 1997 (expected mid-2000) **Title** Day hospitals for people with psychiatric disorders **Review type** Cochrane protocol **Objectives** To determine effectiveness of: day hospital treatment (DHT)	**Search strategy** Electronic Searches of: Cochrane Schizophrenia Group, CINHAL (1982-1997), EMBASE (1980-1997) MEDLINE (1966-1997), PsycLIT (1974-1997) Sociofile (1973-1977) were searched for relevant trials. Further references were sought from published trials. **Quality assessment** Two independent reviewers rated the quality of included trials using categories outlined in the Cochrane Collaboration Handbook. Only trials in category A or B were included in this review. **Statistical analysis** Peto odds ratios (OR) and 95% confidence intervals (CI) for Homogeneous dichotomous data were calculated and a test for heterogeneity was performed. The number needed to treat statistic (NNT), was also calculated. **Quality score (assessed by reviewers):** N/a	**Types of studies** RCTs reporting data on an intention-to-treat basis **Number of studies included** N/a **Years of studies:** N/a **Countries where studies undertaken** N/a	Those with serious mental disorders or illnesses, however defined. Studies were excluded if they were primarily directed at treatment of those with a primary diagnosis of substance abuse or organic brain disease. Studies were also excluded if they were primarily directed at those over the age of 65 or under the age of 18.	Day hospital care or day time attendance at a facility, staffed by dedicated medical and nursing staff, offering the full range of standard psychiatric treatment (from psychiatric assessment and medication to psychological and occupational therapy). The control was standard care, which was defined in four ways: (i) Type 1 where participants are acutely ill = admission to a psychiatric hospital; (ii) Type 2 where participants are recently discharged = out patient follow up; (iii) Type 3 where participants are given more intensive treatment = continuing out patient treatment; and (iv) Type 4, where participants are given long term support = continuing care in hospital.	Outcome measures were grouped into four main categories: numbers maintaining contact with the services; extent of hospital care received; clinical and social outcomes; costs of care.	N/a	N/a

*Cochrane reviews only

Review	Review Methodology	Included trial details	Participants	Intervention details	Outcomes	Results	Author's conclusions
Author Bond et al[44] **Date published (date last updated)*** 1997 **Title** An update on supported employment for people with severe mental Illness **Review type** non-Cochrane **Objectives** To examine the effectiveness of supported employment for people with severe mental illness.	**Search strategy** Manual searches of rehabilitation literature, Psych Abstracts and Index Medicus; computerised searches of dissertation abstracts; and searches of bibliographies, conference proceedings, and listings of federally funded studies were undertaken. Studies had to have been completed by 1995 to be included in the review. **Quality assessment** Not stated **Statistical analysis** Narrative summary. Studies were combined according to study design and a qualitative overview presented. **Quality score (assessed by reviewers): 4**	**Types of studies** Pre-post studies, surveys, quasi-experimental, RCTs and non-RCTs **Number of studies included** Eleven non-experimental studies (7 pre-post studies (n=663); 3 surveys (n=457); 1 quasi-experimental (n=unclear)). Six experimental (1 randomised (n=74); 5 non-RCTs (n=679)). **Years of studies:** 1988-1995 **Countries where studies undertaken** All experimental studies were undertaken in the USA (others not stated)	People with a severe mental illness	Vocational programmes offering supported employment. Programme models included job coaches, assertive community treatment, individual placements and support, day treatment, prevocational training before supported employment, clubhouse, skills training, sheltered workshops and 'choose-get-keep'.	Employment rate, generally reported as the percentage of clients admitted to a programme who actually obtain a paid community job. 'Interval' rates (the percentage of clients obtaining employment at any time during a time interval) and 'status' rates (the percentage of clients currently employed at a fixed interval after programme admission) are also reported.	All studies suggested significant gains in obtaining employment for persons enrolled in a supported employment programme. The experimental studies demonstrated a mean of 58% of clients in supported employment programmes achieving competitive employment, compared with 21% for the control groups, who typically received traditional vocational services. Outcomes relating to time employed and employment earnings also favoured clients in supported employment over control subjects. No evidence was found that suggested that supported employment led to stress levels precipitating higher rehospitalisation rates.	Supported employment appears to be a promising approach for people with severe mental illness, but more studies are needed, with close attention to programme implementation and long-term follow-up.

*Cochrane reviews only

Review	Review Methodology	Included trial details	Participants	Intervention details	Outcomes	Results	Author's conclusions
Author Brooker et al[25] **Date published (date last updated)*** 1996 **Title** The effectiveness of community mental health nursing: a review **Review type** non-Cochrane **Objectives** To examine the effectiveness of community mental health nursing interventions	**Search strategy** MEDLINE, EMBASE, PsycLIT, CINAHL, RCN Nurse-ROM, Science Citation Index, Social Science Citation Index, DHSS-DATA and ASSIA. Cochrane Database of systematic reviews, NHS DARE and NEED databases were searched for relevant trials. Manual searches of the International Nursing Index, and a community mental health nursing bibliography were also undertaken. **Quality assessment** A 5 point scale was used based on Cochrane Collaboration guidelines. This scale assessed the quality of randomisation, whether a power calculation was used, the completeness of follow-up, the length of follow-up, and whether there was blinded assessment of outcomes. **Statistical analysis** Narrative summary **Quality score (assessed by reviewers):** 5	**Types of studies** RCTs and quasi-RCTs **Number of studies included** 10 studies with over 670 participants (for one study the number of patients is not given). **Years of studies:** 1980-1994 **Countries where studies undertaken** All UK based (inclusion criteria was that all had to been UK based)	Individuals with mental health problems, including phobia, obsessional problems, depression, self-harmers, problem drinkers, chronic neurotic disorders and serious mental illness	Community mental health nursing interventions including behavioural psychotherapy, cognitive group therapy, problem solving therapy, counselling, 'supportive' interventions, and assertive outreach/case-management strategies. Comparison group was control or normal GP care.	A number of different outcomes were assessed, including depression, anxiety, fear, general health, hopelessness, social adjustment and process measures such as service use and consumer views and satisfaction.	Significant gains or improvements were reported in five of the studies on outcomes such as depression, self-esteem and general health. Consumer satisfaction also increased in three studies in the groups receiving intervention. Only five of the included studies gave information about the process of randomisation and none of the studies reported using a power calculation.	Little evidence of the effectiveness of community mental health nursing interventions exists and the quality of such evidence is questionable. Those areas of work in which most community mental health nurses are involved are not evaluated.

*Cochrane reviews only

Review	Review Methodology	Included trial details	Participants	Intervention details	Outcomes	Results	Author's conclusions
Author Burns et al33 **Date published (date last updated)*** Ongoing **Title** A systematic review of home treatment compared with admission for mental health problems evaluated in terms of clinical, social, and cost outcomes, user and carer acceptability and sustainability of programmes **Review type** Unpublished **Objectives** To identify trials of community care as an alternative to admission for the severely mentally ill	**Search strategy** CINAHL, EMBASE, The Cochrane Schizophrenia Group's Register (1997), MEDLINE, PsycLIT will be searched for trials **Quality assessment** Quality of the trials will be assessed using the three quality categories outlined in the Cochrane Collaboration Handbook **Statistical analysis** Not clear **Quality score (assessed by reviewers):** check	**Types of studies** Controlled trials **Number of studies included** 91 studies (56 RCTs and 35 non-RCTs) **Years of studies:** Not stated **Countries where studies undertaken** Not stated	People with a severe mental illness	Community or home based care as an alternative to admission that do not readily fall within Case Management, ACT or Crisis Intervention	Hospital days	Meta-analysis with heterogeneous groups of studies is problematic. The evidence bas for the effectiveness of services identifiable as 'home treatment' is not strong. There was some evidence that regularly visiting at home and taking responsibility for both health and social care were associated with reduced hospitalisation. Evidence for other components was inconclusive. The attempt to analyse service utilisation was severely hampered by lack of available data. The conclusion that can be drawn from it are minimal/	No firm conclusions can be drawn concerning the effectiveness of home treatment or its cost-effectiveness, due to the heterogeneity and lack of clarity of control services, range of hospitalisation outcomes and unavailability of standard deviations on mean hospital days data. Questions could therefore be raised concerning the value of meta-analysis in this area.

*Cochrane reviews only

Review	Review Methodology	Included trial details	Participants	Intervention details	Outcomes	Results	Author's conclusions
Author Catty et al[37] **Date published (date last updated)*** 1999 (expected mid-2000) **Title** Day centres for severe mental illness **Review type** Cochrane protocol **Objectives** To determine the effects of day centre care for people with severe mental illness compared to standard community mental health team care and day hospital care	**Search strategy** Allied and Complementary Medicine Database (1985 - 1999), The British Nursing Index (1994 - 1998), The Cochrane Library, EMBASE (1980- 1999), MEDLINE (1966- 1999), PsycLIT (1887-1999), The Royal College of Nurses Database (1985-1996), Sociological Abstracts (1963-1999) The references of all identified studies were also inspected for more studies. The first author of each included study was contacted for information regarding unpublished trials. **Quality assessment** Reviewers will independently rate the quality of all included trials using the Jadad Scale. Only trials reliably rating over two on this scale will be included. **Statistical analysis** Peto Odds Ratio with 95% confidence intervals will be estimated and a test of heterogeneity performed. Where possible, the number needed to treat statistic (NNT) will also calculated. **Quality score (assessed by reviewers)**: N/a	**Types of studies** RCTs comparing day centres with standard care or day hospital care. **Number of studies included** N/a **Years of studies:** N/a **Countries where studies undertaken** N/a	Adults with a severe mental illness such as schizophrenia or other psychotic illnesses	Day centre care: defined as day time attendance at a non-medical services day setting, excluding specialist work units or crisis facilities. The comparison was standard care which was defined as the care offered as standard to people in the community. The effects of standard community mental health team care and day hospital care were not a focus of the review.	Death, suicide or natural causes; leaving the study early; clinical response (relapse, change in global state or in psychotic symptoms); violent or criminal behaviour; service use (hospital admission, days in hospital); economic outcomes; quality of life / satisfaction with care for either recipients of care or carers	N/a	N/a

*Cochrane reviews only

Review	Author	Review Methodology	Included trial details	Participants	Intervention details	Outcomes	Results	Author's conclusions
Author Crowther et al[46] **Date published (date last updated)*** 1999 (expected mid-2000) **Title** Vocational rehabilitation for people with severe mental disorders **Review type** Cochrane protocol **Objectives** To determine the effects of vocational rehabilitation services for helping people with severe mental disorders to obtain employment		**Search strategy** CINAHL (1982 - 1998), EMBASE (1980 - 1998), MEDLINE (1966 - 1998), PsycLIT (1987 - 1998) will be searched for relevant trials. All reviews identified by the search above will be examined to determine if any studies have not been detected. **Quality assessment** Both reviewers will rate the quality of all included studies based on the three quality categories outlined in the Cochrane Collaboration Handbook. All trials in category A B or C were included in the review. **Statistical analysis** Relative risks (RR) and 95% confidence intervals (CI) will be calculated for dichotomous outcomes and an intention to treat analysis will be undertaken. **Quality score (assessed by reviewers):** N/a	**Types of studies** RCTs **Number of studies included** N/a **Years of studies:** N/a **Countries where studies undertaken** N/a	Adults suffering from severe mental disorder defined as schizophrenia and schizophrenia-like disorders; bipolar disorder; or depression with psychotic features	Three types of vocational rehabilitation were defined. 1. Approaches involving (i) pre-vocational training (including the traditional and 'clubhouse' approaches 2. Approaches involving immediate placement (i.e. supported employment) 3. Approaches involving an enhancement of either a pre-vocational or immediate placement approach.	The primary outcome will be the number of people in competitive employment at the end of the study. Secondary outcome include: other employment outcomes; clinical and social outcomes and costs	N/a	N/a

*Cochrane reviews only

Review	Review Methodology	Included trial details	Participants	Intervention details	Outcomes	Results	Author's conclusions
Author Drake et al[40] **Date published (date last updated)*** 1998 **Title** Review of integrated mental health and substance abuse treatment for patients with dual disorders **Review type** non-Cochrane **Objectives** To describe the evolution of integrated treatment programmes and to review the research to date on these programmes	**Search strategy** MEDLINE and Project Cork databases were searched and project officers at several relevant agencies were contacted **Quality assessment** Not stated **Statistical analysis** Narrative summary **Quality score (assessed by reviewers):** 5	**Types of studies** Controlled and uncontrolled trials **Number of studies included** 36 studies (23 uncontrolled, 6 quasi-experimental, and 7 experimental; total number of participants not stated) **Years of studies:** 1986-1997 **Countries where studies undertaken** Not stated	People dually diagnosed with severe mental illness (such as schizophrenia) and substance use disorder (alcohol or other drugs)	Integrated treatments that combined mental health and substance abuse treatments consisting of psychosocial interventions, as distinguished from pharmacological therapies. In the review, the interventions were divided into four categories: dual-disorders treatment groups (4 studies); intensive integrated treatments (9 studies); Community Support Programmes (CSP) demonstration projects for young adults with co-occurring disorders (13 studies); and comprehensive integrated dual-disorders programmes (10 studies).	Engagement in treatment, substance use behaviours and outcomes, hospital utilisation and symptoms of mental illness	Treatment groups, intensive integrated treatments and CSP demonstration projects were limited by poor methodology, and results were inconsistent. Although the studies of comprehensive integrated dual-disorders programmes were limited in different ways, the results provided encouraging evidence for the effectiveness of integrated treatment of dual disorders. Integrated treatment, especially when delivered for 18 months or longer, resulted in significant reductions of substance abuse and, in some cases, in substantial rates of readmission as well as reduction in hospital use and/or improvements in other outcomes.	Given the magnitude and severity of the problem of dual disorders, more controlled research on integrated treatment is needed.

*Cochrane reviews only

Review	Review Methodology	Included trial details	Participants	Intervention details	Outcomes	Results	Author's conclusions
Author Hayes and Macdonald[5] **Date published (date last updated)*** 1997 (expected mid-2000) **Title** Supported housing for people with severe mental disorders **Review type** Cochrane protocol **Objectives** To determine the effectiveness, including cost-effectiveness, of supported housing schemes and outreach support schemes for people in with severe mental disorder living in the community	**Search strategy** The Cochrane Schizophrenia Group's Register and the Cochrane Library will be searched. Citation searching will be undertaken electronically. Social Citation Index and Science Citation Index will be searched for both included and excluded studies. **Quality assessment** Two independent reviewers will rate the quality of included trials based on the three categories outlined in the Cochrane Collaboration Handbook. Only studies assigned to categories A and B will be selected. **Statistical analysis** OR will be calculated, and a test for heterogeneity performed **Quality score (assessed by reviewers):** N/a	**Types of studies** RCTs. Quasi-randomized trials will also be identified for a sensitivity analysis. **Number of studies included** N/a **Years of studies:** N/a **Countries where studies undertaken**	People with 'severe mental disorders' however diagnosed, including those with multiple diagnoses, who are living alone or with a partner and/or children but not living with their parents or extended family	Supported housing schemes or outreach support schemes. The comparison was standard care, which was defined as the normal level of psychiatric care provided in the area where the trial was conducted.	1. Service utilisation Evicted from tenancy; hospitalisation; imprisoned; and psychiatric service contact. 2. Medical/mental state changes, death (including suicide); general mental state; self-esteem; and specific symptoms including well-being. 3. Satisfaction Professional support workers' satisfaction; and tenant or respondent satisfaction. 4. Social functioning employment status; and general social function. 5. Quality of life, general quality of life. 6. Economic	N/a	N/a

*Cochrane reviews only

Review	Review Methodology	Included trial details	Participants	Intervention details	Outcomes	Results	Author's conclusions
Author Henderson et al[35] **Date published (date last updated)*** 1999 **Title** Patient held clinical information for people with psychotic illnesses **Review type** Cochrane review **Objectives** To evaluate the effects of personalised and accessible patient-held clinical information for people with a diagnosis of psychotic illness	**Search strategy** AMED, Biological Abstracts, British Nursing Index, CAB, CINAHL, The Cochrane Controlled Trials Register, EMBASE, HealthStar, HMIC (King's Fund Database & HELMIS), MEDLINE, PsycLIT, Royal College of Nursing Database, SIGLE, Sociological Abstracts and the Internet were searched for relevant trials. This was supplemented by personal contact with the Executive Board of the European Network for Mental Health Service Evaluation. **Quality assessment** Two reviewers will independently rate the quality of all included studies based on the three quality categories outlined in the Cochrane Collaboration Handbook **Statistical analysis** For binary outcomes a standard estimation of the risk ratio (RR) and its 95% confidence interval (CI) was calculated. The number needed to treat statistic (NNT) was also calculated. **Quality score (assessed by reviewers)**: 7	**Types of studies** RCTs and quasi-RCTs **Number of studies included** None **Years of studies:** N/a **Countries where studies undertaken** N/a	Adults with a diagnosis of a psychotic illness. Although the main focus of this review was those with schizophrenia and schizophrenia-like disorders those with other psychoses such as bipolar disorder and depression with psychotic features were also of interest. People whose main problem and primary diagnosis was one of deliberate self-harm were not the focus of this review.	Patient-held information: any personalised and accessible clinical information held by the patient beyond standard care. This includes both patient-held records (notes made by professionals at appointments and kept by the patient) and crisis cards (personal information held for use in the event of a crisis or relapse). Generic information on diagnosis, treatment or services available was excluded. The comparison was standard information which was defined as any information routinely held such as appointment cards and generic information on diagnosis, treatment or services available. In certain settings standard information may include a copy of the treatment plan with contact details for the key carers.	Primary outcomes were 1. Hospital admission 2. Death from causes other than suicide 3. Violence to self or others Secondary outcome measures 1. Rates of criminal charges 2. Mental state 3. Satisfaction with health care 4. Perceived coercion on hospital admission 5. Acceptability of management as measured by loss to follow up within the study 6. Compliance with treatment other than the intervention 7. Social functioning 8. Economic costs of all care and health care 9. Other relevant measures	Not one study met the inclusion criteria for the review. One study was found on the use of client held records for people with long term mental illness but the participants had not been randomised. Two important randomised studies are ongoing.	There is a gap in the evidence regarding patient-held, personalised, accessible clinical information for people with psychotic illnesses. It cannot be assumed that patient-held information is beneficial or cost-effective without evidence from well planned, conducted and reported randomised trials.

*Cochrane reviews only

Review	Review Methodology	Included trial details	Participants	Intervention details	Outcomes	Results	Author's conclusions
Author Holloway et al[26] **Date published (date last updated)*** 1995 **Title** Case management - a critical review of the outcome literature **Review type** non-Cochrane **Objectives** To examine the effect of case management (care management) on psychiatric patients	**Search strategy** APA PsycLIT CD-ROM system (from 1987-March 1993 wasseached for relevant trials. Citations in the literature were identified and the authors also used their knowledge of the field. **Quality assessment** Study characteristics (study design, number of subjects, inclusion criteria, follow-up period) were listed in a table **Statistical analysis** Narrative summary **Quality score (assessed by reviewers):** 4	**Types of studies** RCTs, matched-control, repeated measures (own-control), and descriptive studies **Number of studies included** 23 studies with a total of 3,803 participants (including 11 RCTs with a total of 1,634 participants) **Years of studies:** 1980-1995 **Countries where studies undertaken** USA: 16 UK: 3 Canada: 2 Australia: 7 Germany: 7	People with psychiatric disorder or disability. Generally, patients with organic brain disorder or primary diagnosis of alcohol or drug dependence were excluded.	Brokerage case management - focusing on the organisation and co-ordination of services on behalf of the client. Clinical case management - assertive community treatment, the psychosocial rehabilitation model and the strengths model.	The number of hospital days, the number of admissions, the costs of case management, use of community care services, satisfaction with services, quality of life, symptoms, social functioning, family burden, social networks/ relationships	*Hospital utilisation (21 studies)*: a significant decrease in the number of hospital days is reported in 11 studies. Number of admissions decreased significantly in 7 studies. *Compliance (9 studies)*: 6 studies showed an improvement in the case management (CM) group. *Changes in symptomatology (8 studies)*: 4 studies found no significant difference between groups and 4 studies found a decrease in symptomatology in CM group. *Overall functioning (8 studies)*: 2 studies showed an improvement in CM group. *Burden on families (3 studies)*: 3 studies found the burden on the families of patients receiving CM type services were not increased.	Case management practice can have some impact on patients' use of services (including marked decrease in hospital stay); satisfaction with services; engagement with services; and social networks and relationships when it is delivered as a direct, clinical service with high staff:patient ratios. Different models of case management need to be compared.

*Cochrane reviews only

Review	Review Methodology	Included trial details	Participants	Intervention details	Outcomes	Results	Author's conclusions
Author Johnstone and Zolese[36] **Date published (date last updated)*** 1999 **Title** Systematic review of the effectiveness of planned short hospital stays for mental health care **Review type** Cochrane review and published review. Results taken from published review **Objectives** To determine the effect of planned short stay admission policies versus a long or standard stay for people with serious mental illnesses	**Search strategy** Biological Abstracts (1982-1995), Cochrane Schizophrenia Group's Register (December 1998), EMBASE (1980-1998), MEDLINE (1966-1998) and PsycLIT (1974-1995) were searched for relevant trials. Further references were sought from published trials and their authors. **Quality assessment** Both reviewers rated the quality of all included studies using three quality categories as described in the Cochrane Collaboration Handbook. Only trials categorised as A or B were included. **Statistical analysis** Peto odds ratios (OR) and 95% confidence intervals were calculated and a test for heterogeneity was performed. Excluded data from results based on information from less than 50% of the original participants. Analysis was on an intention to treat. **Quality score (assessed by reviewers):** 7	**Types of studies** RCTs **Number of studies included** Four RCTs with a total of 628 participants **Years of studies:** 1975-1979 **Countries where studies undertaken** USA: 3 UK: 1	Those suffering from schizophrenia, related disorders or 'severe/chronic mental disorders/illnesses', however diagnosed	Planned short stay/brief admission - however defined within the studies. The comparison was long stay or standard care - however defined within the studies.	Relapse; readmission; death (suicides and all causes); violent incidents (self, others, property); lost to follow up; premature discharge; delayed discharge; mental state (not improved); social functioning; patient satisfaction, quality of life, self esteem, and psychological wellbeing; family burden; imprisonment; employment status; independent living; total cost of care; and average length of hospital stay.	Patients allocated to planned short hospital stays had no more readmissions (in four trials, OR 0.93, 95% CI: 0.66 to 1.29 with no heterogeneity), no more losses to follow up (in three trials of 404 patients, 1.09, 0.62 to 1.91 no heterogeneity), and more successful discharges on time (in three trials of 404 patients, 0.47, 0.27 to 0.85) than patients allocated long hospital stays or standard care. Some evidence showed that patients allocated planned short hospital stay were no more likely to leave hospital prematurely and had a greater chance of being employed than those allocated long hospital stay or standard care. Data on mental, social, and family outcomes not summated. There were few or no data on deaths, patient satisfaction, violence, criminal behaviour & costs.	The effectiveness of care in mental hospitals is important to patients, carers, and policy makers. Despite inadequacies in the data, this review suggests that planned short hospital stays do not encourage a "revolving door" pattern of care for people with serious mental illness and may be more effective than standard care. Further pragmatic trials are needed on the most effective organisation and delivery of care in mental hospitals.

*Cochrane reviews only

Review	Review Methodology	Included trial details	Participants	Intervention details	Outcomes	Results	Author's conclusions
Author Joy et al[34] **Date published (date last updated)*** 2000 (February 2000) **Title** Crisis intervention for people with severe mental illnesses **Review type** Cochrane review **Objectives** To review the effects of a crisis intervention model for anyone with serious mental illness experiencing an acute episode, compared to 'standard care'	**Search strategy** Biological Abstracts (1985-1998), CINAHL (1982-1998), The Cochrane Library, the Cochrane Schizophrenia Register of trials, EMBASE (1980-1998), MEDLINE (1966-1998), PsycLIT (1974-1998), Sociofile (1974-1998) and the ISI database (Science Citations and Social Science Citations) were all searched for relevant trials. Further references were sought from published trials and their authors. **Quality assessment** Two reviewers independently rated the quality of all included studies using the Jadad scale and the Cochrane Collaboration Handbook. Only trials reliably rating over 2 on this scale were included. **Statistical analysis** Where possible OR were calculated and an intention-to-treat was undertaken. Tests of heterogeneity were undertaken. **Quality score (assessed by reviewers):** 7	**Types of studies** RCTs **Number of studies included** Five RCTs with a total of 764 participants **Years of studies:** 1964-1994 **Countries where studies undertaken** Canada: 1 Australia: 1 UK: 1 USA: 2	Anyone with schizophrenia or other serious mental illness (however diagnosed), presenting to or referred to a social/psychiatric/ nursing service because they were experiencing a psychosocial crisis (however defined). People in crisis with drug-induced psychosis or in a depressive crisis were excluded.	Crisis Intervention defined as any type of crisis-orientated treatment of an acute psychiatric episode by staff with a specific remit to deal with such situations, in and beyond 'office hours'. The comparison was standard care which was defined as the normal care given to those suffering from acute psychiatric episodes in the area concerned. Studies comparing different models of 'crisis intervention', mobile and non-mobile units, were also utilised in a second comparison within this review.	Hospitalisation; patient, carer and staff satisfaction with treatment; clinical outcomes (death/suicide, improvement, compliance with medication, antipsychotic medication relapses); social functioning and economic cost of treatment and health care.	Home care crisis interventions were slightly superior in avoiding repeat admissions (OR 0.63 95% CI 0.42 - 0.94). This result is not robust due to heterogeneity. Home care reduces loss to follow-up at 6 (OR 0.62, 95% CI 0.42-0.91) and 12 months (0.65, 95% CI 0.44-0.96), reduces family burden (OR 0.20, 95% CI 0.10-0.42) and is a more satisfactory form of care for both patients and families. No differences in loss, death or mental state were found. All studies found home care to be more cost effective than hospital care but all data were either skewed or unusable. No data on staff satisfaction, carer input, compliance with medication and number of relapses were available.	The five included studies evaluated crisis interventions as part of home care programmes for acutely ill people, rather than 'pure' crisis interventions. Home care crisis interventions were found to be superior to standard hospital care in promoting greater acceptance of treatment. It may also be a more economical option.

*Cochrane reviews only

Review	Review Methodology	Included trial details	Participants	Intervention details	Outcomes	Results	Author's conclusions
Author Latimer [31] **Date published (date last updated)*** 1999 **Title** Economic impacts of assertive community treatment: a review of the literature **Review type** non-Cochrane **Objectives** To focus on economic issues associated with the assertive community treatment (ACT) model	**Search strategy** A literature search was undertaken (databases and years not specified) and experts were contacted **Quality assessment** Not stated, although details of study design and fidelity to the ACT model were assessed **Statistical analysis** Multiple-regression methods were used to relate reduction in hospital days to program fidelity and other contextual factors **Quality score (assessed by reviewers):** 3	**Types of studies** RCTs, pre-post studies and quasi-experimental (non-random controlled) studies **Number of studies included** 19 RCTs with a total of 3,652 participants, and 15 non-RCTs with a total of 1,139 participants **Years of studies:** 1980-1998 **Countries where studies undertaken** USA: 28 Australia: 4 Sweden: 1 UK: 1	People with a severe mental illness	Assertive community treatment. Programmes were coded as being of 'high fidelity' if, in addition to following a shared-caseload model and providing the majority of services in the community, they explicitly met at least 4 of the following 5 criteria: 1) staff:client ratio of 1:12 or better; 2) a psychiatrist on staff; 3) at least one nurse on staff; 4) at least some coverage outside of normal working hours; 5) at least two team meetings every week. Programmes were coded as being of 'medium fidelity' if they explicitly met at least 4 Criteria and as 'low fidelity' if they met less than 2 criteria.	Time spent in hospital and costs (to be reported in review of cost-effectiveness)	High fidelity programmes appeared to reduce hospital days by about 23 percentage points more than lower-fidelity programmes (95% CI: -41.2, 5.2). The estimated regression coefficients imply that a high-fidelity program reduces hospitalisations by about 58% over I year if the alternative involves some type of case management and by 78% if it does not. ACT appears to increase the proportion of clients who live in independent housing situations, but the effect on use of supervised housing, and therefore on housing costs, is ambiguous. The effects on use of most other resources are inconsistent across studies.	The most reliable cost offset to ACT treatment costs appears to be reduced hospital use. Using Quebec costs, an ACT program must enrol people with prior hospital use of about 50 days yearly, on average, to break even. As care systems evolve to reduce their reliance on hospitalisation as a care modality with or without ACT, this threshold will became increasingly difficult to achieve. The primary justification for implementing ACT services will then become their clinical benefits.

*Cochrane reviews only

Review	Review Methodology	Included trial details	Participants	Intervention details	Outcomes	Results	Author's conclusions
Author Lees et al[42] **Date published (date last updated)*** 1999 **Title** Therapeutic community effectiveness: a systematic international review of therapeutic community treatment for people with personality disorders and mentally disordered offenders **Review type** non-Cochrane **Objectives** To review the international literature on the effectiveness of therapeutic communities with such client groups.	**Search strategy** 26 electronic databases were searched, as well as journal citations, books, grey literature, conference proceedings, and hand-searching. There were no language restrictions. **Quality assessment** Studies were categorised according to their level of resolution, or their position on the research methodolgy hierachy. **Statistical analysis** Summary odds ratios, 5% and I were calculated for all controlled trials. Studies were also subdivided into RCTs, and types of therapeutic interventions. **Quality score (assessed by reviewers)**: 5	**Types of studies** All types of post-treatment outcome studies with a control **Number of studies included** 52 controlled studies of which 10 were RCTs (total number of participants not stated) **Years of studies:** Not stated **Countries where studies undertaken** Not stated, but most were undertaken in the UK or USA	People with personality disorders, mentally disordered offenders, and substance abusers	Therapeutic community described as 'a consciously-designed social environment and programme within a residential or day unit in which the social and group process is harnessed with therapeutic intent. In the therapeutic community the community is the primary therapeutic instrument.' Also included were hierarchical, or concept-based therapeutic communities. These are usually for substance abusers, in both secure and non-secure settings, both psychiatric and non-psychiatric, although there are considerably more in the USA, Canada, and other parts of the world than in the UK.	Outcomes as described in the studies. These included interpersonal relationships, behaviour, self-esteem, and other social and psychological outcomes. The meta-analysis was based on the effectiveness of the treatment, but the outcome was not described.	29 studies were included in the meta-analysis. The OR for effectiveness for all 29 studies was 0.57 ((5% CI: 0.52 to 0.61). The OR for RCTs only was 0.47 (95% CI: 0.39 to 0.55). The OR for democratic therapeutic communities was 0.695 (95% CI: 0.631 to 0.769). The OR for secure therapeutic communities was 0.54 (95% CI: 0.50 to 0.60). The OR for concept therapeutic communities was 0.32 (95% CI: 0.27 to 0.37).	Therapeutic communities have not produced the amount or quality of research literature, given the length of time they have been in existence, and the quality of staff we know exists and has existed in therapeutic communities. The meta-analysis indicates that existing research is in favour of therapeutic communities. There should be more, and more good quality, and comparative, research on therapeutic communities, in order to confirm the case that therapeutic communities are effective.

*Cochrane reviews only

Review	Review Methodology	Included trial details	Participants	Intervention details	Outcomes	Results	Author's conclusions
Author Lart et al[41] **Date published (date last updated)*** 1999 **Title** Women and secure psychiatric services: a literature review **Review type** Non-Cochrane **Objectives** To examine the evidence for effectiveness and efficiency of different service delivery models for women in secure psychiatric services.	**Search strategy** The following databases were searched: MEDLINE (1972 to June 1997), EMBASE (1980 to 1997), PsycLIT (1972 to June 1997), Sociofile (1974 to June 1997), Cochrane Library(1997 issue 3), SIGLE (Blaiseline On-line), Mental Health Abstracts (DIALOG On-line). The search terms were provided. Calls for information were sent to government departments, professional Organisations, relevant agencies and key researchers and authors. **Quality assessment** Not stated. **Statistical analysis** Not applicable, as only one relevant study was found. **Quality score (assessed by reviewers):** 6	**Types of studies** Initially, all studies which provided information on short, medium or long-term outcomes of interventions in services for women assessed as needing psychiatric care in conditions of security were included. **Number of studies included** One cohort study, (n=33). **Years of studies:** Not stated **Countries where studies undertaken** Not stated	Women admitted for secure psychiatric care.	Interventions/regimes in services for women assessed as needing psychiatric care in conditions of security.	A "subjective rating" (as defined by the authors of the study concerned) of progress, based on subsequent psychiatric condition, behaviour in and out of hospital or prison, work record, further court appearances and hospital re-admissions.	Of the 33 women included, 32 women were followed up (one escaped). Of these, 18 were given a rating of "poor" outcome, and 14 one of "good" outcome. The group of woman admitted from other psychiatric hospitals, particularly those admitted following violence in hospital, tended to have poorer outcomes than those admitted from the courts. Outcome was not related to length of stay.	Only one study was identified examining the effectiveness of psychiatric care. This study found a poorer outcome amongst women admitted from psychiatric hospital compared with women admitted from courts.

*Cochrane reviews only

Review	Review Methodology	Included trial details	Participants	Intervention details	Outcomes	Results	Author's conclusions
Author Lehman et al[45] **Date published (date last updated)*** 1995 **Title** Vocational rehabilitation in schizophrenia **Review type** non-Cochrane **Objectives** To determine if vocational rehabilitation interventions enhance the outcomes of persons with schizophrenia	**Search strategy** PsycLIT and MEDLINE from 1966-1993 were searched for relevant trials. Reviews were included in this search. **Quality assessment** Number of patients diagnosed with schizophrenia and information about the relationship of diagnosis to intervention impacts. **Statistical analysis** Narrative summary **Quality score (assessed by reviewers):** 3	**Types of studies** Controlled trials **Number of studies included** 24 trials with a total of 2,715 participants. **Years of studies:** 1963 -1995 **Countries where studies undertaken** Not stated	People with schizophrenia	Vocational rehabilitation, sheltered workshops, employment or employment supported, rehabilitation counselling, assertive community treatment (ACT) and job developer.	Vocational functioning	Vocational rehabilitation enhances employment rates for patients whiles they are on these programmes (but not after leaving the programmes). Supportive employment closely co-ordinated with clinical care can enhance the rate of competitive employment amongst these patients. Vocational interventions are associated with reduced hospital admissions.	Vocational rehabilitation programs generally have a positive influence on work-related activities, but most have failed to show substantial and enduring impacts on independent, competitive employment. Supported employment suggests that vocational rehabilitation offers greater promise than do transitional and sheltered employment approaches. Vocational rehabilitation may also positively influence medication compliance, symptom reduction, and relapse.

*Cochrane reviews only

Review	Review Methodology	Included trial details	Participants	Intervention details	Outcomes	Results	Author's conclusions
Author Ley et al[39] **Date published (date last updated)*** 1999 **Title** Treatment programmes for people with both severe mental illness and substance misuse **Review type** Cochrane review **Objectives** To evaluate the effectiveness of treatment programmes within psychiatric care for people with problems of both substance misuse and serious mental illness	**Search strategy** Biological Abstracts (1985-1998), CINAHL (1982-1998), The Cochrane Library (Issue 3, 1998), The Cochrane Schizophrenia Group's Register of trials (August 1998), EMBASE (1980-1998), MEDLINE (1966-1998), PsycLIT (1974-1998) and Sociofile (1974-1998) were searched for relevant trials. Citations of all trials were searched and further studies sought from published trials and their authors. **Quality assessment** Trials were allocated to the three categories described in the Cochrane Collaboration Handbook and the Jadad scale **Statistical analysis** For binary data the initial analysis was the estimation of the Peto odds ratios (OR) and the 95% Confidence Interval (CI). Data from studies where attrition was greater than 50% were not used because of the strong likelihood of bias. **Quality score (assessed by reviewers): 7**	**Types of studies** RCTs **Number of studies included** Six RCTs with a total of 659 participants **Years of studies:** 1991-1998 **Countries where studies undertaken** All were undertaken in the USA	Any individual presenting to adult psychiatric services with severe mental illness (however diagnosed) and current problems of substance misuse (however diagnosed). People with serious affective disorders, such as manic-depressive illness, were included if it was impossible to extricate their data from the rest. If possible, those with organic disorder, personality disorder and those who solely abused tobacco were excluded.	Any programmes of substance misuse treatment within standard psychiatric care. This included serial, parallel and integrated treatment programmes. The comparison was no specific substance misuse treatment programme within standard psychiatric care. Standard psychiatric care should be stated to be the normal level of psychiatric care in the area where the trial was conducted.	Primary outcomes: 1. numbers lost to treatment 2. symptoms of severe mental illness 3. substance use 4. hospitalisation Other secondary outcomes were: 1. death (all causes) 2. violence to others 3. quality of life 4. patient satisfaction 5. carer satisfaction 6. social functioning 7. homelessness; 8. employment 9. average change in social functioning.	Six relevant studies, four of which were small, were identified. In general, the quality of design and reporting was not high. Clinically important outcomes such as relapse of severe mental illness, violence to others, patient or carer satisfaction, social functioning and employment were not reported. There is no clear evidence supporting an advantage of any type of substance misuse programme for those with serious mental illness over the value of standard care. No one programme is clearly superior to another.	The current momentum for integrated programmes is not based on good evidence. Implementation of new specialist substance misuse services for those with serious mental illnesses should be within the context of simple, well designed controlled clinical trials.

*Cochrane reviews only

Review	Review Methodology	Included trial details	Participants	Intervention details	Outcomes	Results	Author's conclusions
Author Marshall & Lockwood[30] **Date published (date last updated)*** 1998 (25 February) **Title** Assertive community treatment for people with severe mental disorders **Review type** Cochrane review **Objectives** To determine the effectiveness of Assertive Community Treatment (ACT) as an alternative to i. standard community care, ii. traditional hospital-based rehabilitation, and iii. case management	**Search strategy** CINAHL (1982-1997), the Cochrane Schizophrenia Group's Register of trials (1997), EMBASE (1980-1997), MEDLINE (1966-1997), PsycLIT (1974-1997) and SCISEARCH (1997) were all searched for relevant trials. References of all identified studies were searched for further trial citations. **Quality assessment** Both reviewers rated the quality of all included trials. A rating was given for each trial based on the three quality categories as described in the Cochrane Collaboration Handbook. Only trials in category A or B were included in this review. All included trials were to be conducted on an intention-to-treat basis. **Statistical analysis** Peto Odds Ratios (OR) and the number needed to treat (NNT) were calculated. **Quality score (assessed by reviewers): 7**	**Types of studies** RCTs **Number of studies included** 20 (3502 participants) **Years of studies:** 1973-1997 **Countries where studies undertaken** USA: 16 Canada: 2 Sweden: 1 UK: 1	The majority were adults (16-85) suffering from severe mental disorder. Individuals with substance abuse and without a severe mental disorder were excluded.	All interventions described in trial reports as 'Assertive Community Treatment', 'Assertive Case Management' or 'PACT', or as being based on the Madison, Treatment in Community Living, Assertive Community Treatment or Stein and Tests models. Trials which did not meet the criteria for ACT were considered in the Case Management review. The present review excluded home-based care and studies which considered the use of ACT as an alternative to acute hospital admission.	Remaining in contact with the psychiatric services, extent of psychiatric hospital admissions, clinical and social outcome and costs	Those receiving ACT are more likely to remain in contact with services than people receiving standard community care (OR 0.51, 99% CI 037-0.70). This group also experienced fewer hospital admissions (OR 0.59, 99% CI 0.41-0.85) and had shorter time in hospital. Individuals receiving ACT were less likely to be homeless or unemployed, more likely to be living independently and more satisfied than patients receiving standard care. There were no differences in deaths, imprisonment /arrests/police contacts, mental state, social functioning and quality of life. While ACT reduced the costs of hospital care, it did not have a clear cut advantage when other costs were taken into account.	ACT is a clinically effective approach to managing the care of severely mentally ill people in the community. ACT, if correctly targeted on high users of in-patient care, can substantially reduce the costs of hospital care whilst improving outcome and patient satisfaction.

*Cochrane reviews only

Review	Review Methodology	Included trial details	Participants	Intervention details	Outcomes	Results	Author's conclusions
Author Marshall et al[2] **Date published (date last updated)*** 1997 (December) **Title** Case management for people with severe mental disorders **Review type** Cochrane review **Objectives** To determine the effects of case management for severely mentally ill people in the community compared to standard care	**Search strategy** CINAHL (1997), the Cochrane Schizophrenia Group's Register of trials (1997), EMBASE (1980-1995), MEDLINE (1966-1995), PsycLIT (1974-1995) and SCISEARCH (1997) were all searched for relevant trials. References of all identified studies were searched for further trial citations. **Quality assessment** Two reviewers rated the quality of all included trials using the Cochrane Collaboration Handbook. Only trials in category A or B were included in this review. **Statistical analysis** Odds ratios and the number needed to treat were estimated **Quality score (assessed by reviewers):** 7	**Types of studies** RCTs **Number of studies included** Eleven RCTs (1,642 participants) **Years of studies:** 1985-1997 **Countries where studies undertaken** USA: 6 UK: 4	The majority were adults of working age suffering from severe mental disorder (schizophrenia, bipolar disorder, depression with psychotic features, those with severe mental illness plus substance abuse)	Described as 'case management' in the trial report. The UK terms 'care program approach' and 'care program approach' were treated as synonyms for case management. The review excluded Assertive Community Treatment and Home-Based Care.	Numbers remaining in contact with the psychiatric services; extent of psychiatric hospital admissions; clinical and social outcomes; and costs.	Case management (CM) increased the numbers remaining in contact with services (OR 0.70; 99%CI 0.50-0.98). CM approximately doubled the numbers admitted to psychiatric hospital (OR 1.84; 99% CI 1.33-2.57). Except for a positive finding on compliance, from one study, CM showed no significant advantages over standard care on any psychiatric or social variable. Cost data did not favour case management but insufficient information was available to permit definitive conclusions.	Case management ensures that people remain in contact with psychiatric services but it also increases hospital admission rates. There is some evidence that it improves compliance, but does not produce clinically significant improvement in mental state, social functioning, or quality of life. Case management increases health care costs, although this is not certain.

*Cochrane reviews only

Review	Review Methodology	Included trial details	Participants	Intervention details	Outcomes	Results	Author's conclusions
Author Mueser et al[27] **Date published (date last updated)*** 1998 **Title** Models of community care for severe mental illness: a review of research on case management **Review type** non-Cochrane **Objectives** To review the results of all research studies that sought to evaluate the effectiveness of one or more models of case management	**Search strategy** Relevant articles, presentations, reports to government granting agencies and unpublished papers were identified through literature reviews, searches of computer databases and contact with researchers in the field. **Quality assessment** Details of study design, follow-up period and attrition rates were reported. **Statistical analysis** Narrative summary **Quality score (assessed by reviewers):** 5	**Types of studies** RCTs, controlled and non-controlled studies **Number of studies included** 75 studies (32 RCTs, 18 controlled and 25 pre-post). Total number of participants not stated (range of participant numbers in the studies was 15-873). **Years of studies:** 1973-1990 **Countries where studies undertaken** USA: 27 RCTs + 35 non-controlled studies; UK: 3 RCTs; Australia: 1 RCT and 2 non-controlled studies; Canada: 5 non-controlled studies Sweden: 1 RCT; Germany: 1 non-controlled study	People with severe mental illness	Standard case management (broker and clinical case management), assertive community treatment, intensive case management, strengths case management, rehabilitation case management.	Time in hospital, symptoms, social adjustment, housing stability, jail/arrests, substance abuse, medication compliance, quality of life, vocational functioning, patient satisfaction, relative satisfaction.	Controlled research on assertive community treatment (ACT) and intensive case management (ICM) indicate that these models reduce time in the hospital and improve housing stability, especially among patients who are high service users. ACT and ICM appear to have moderate effects on improving symptomatology and quality of life. Most studies suggest little effect of ACT and ICM on social functioning arrests and time spent in prison. Research on other models is inconclusive.	Directions for future research on models of community care include evaluating implementation fidelity, exploring patient predictors of improvement, and evaluating the role of the helping alliance in mediating outcome.

*Cochrane reviews only

Review	Author	Review Methodology	Included trial details	Participants	Intervention details	Outcomes	Results	Author's conclusions
Author Nicol et al[47] **Date published (date last updated)*** 1998 **Title** Life skills programmes for chronic mental illnesses **Review type** Cochrane review **Objectives** To compare the effectiveness of life skills programmes with standard care for people with chronic mental health problems. Also to compare outcomes for those taking part in life skills programmes of differing duration; in hospital or community settings; with trained/untrained care workers		**Search strategy** CINAHL (1982-1997), The Cochrane Library (Issue 2, 1997), The Cochrane Schizophrenia Group's Register of Trials, EMBASE (1980-1997), MEDLINE (1966-1997) and PsycLIT (1974-1997) were methodically searched. Hand searches and scrutiny of references supplemented this process. **Quality assessment** The quality of methodology of each of included studies was independently rated using the Cochrane Collaboration guideline **Statistical analysis** For dichotomous outcomes, odds ratios and confidence intervals were used. Where possible, as a measure of efficiency, the number needed to treat (NNT) was also calculated. **Quality score (assessed by reviewers):** 7	**Types of studies** RCTs or quasi-RCTs **Number of studies included** Two RCTs with a total of 38 participants **Years of studies:** 1983 **Countries where studies undertaken** Not stated	Adults aged 16-65 with chronic mental illnesses diagnosed by any criteria. Sufferers from dementia were excluded.	Life skills programmes were defined as any group or individual programme involving independent functioning in daily living. These programmes could include training in managing money, organising and running a home, domestic skills and personal self care. Evaluation of specific social skills training was not a focus of this review. Programmes of five sessions and less were considered as 'brief', and six or more as 'other'. Trained staff were those personnel who held a professionally recognised health care qualification. The comparison was standard care which was defined as the normal level of psychiatric care provided in the area where the trial is being carried out.	The primary outcome was self-care functioning at personal and domestic level (life skills). Other outcomes of interest were: 1. Quality of life; 2. Social functioning; 3. Satisfaction with care, whether measured directly or by leaving the study early; 4. Mental state: symptom change, relapse, hospitalisation changes - admitted/discharged; 5. Behaviour: incidents of violence, to self, others and property; 6. Death; and, if available, 7. Economic outcomes. All outcomes are reported for the short term (less than 6 months), medium term (7-12 months) and long term (over 1 year).	Two randomised controlled trials were included with a total of 38 participants. Data were sparse and no clear effects were demonstrated.	If life skills training is to continue as part of rehabilitation programmes a large, well designed, conducted and reported pragmatic randomised trial is an urgent necessity. There may even be an argument for stating that maintenance of current practice, outside of a randomised trial, is unethical.

*Cochrane reviews only

Review	Review Methodology	Included trial details	Participants	Intervention details	Outcomes	Results	Author's conclusions
Author Reda and Makhoul[49] **Date published (date last updated)*** 2000 (expected mid-2001) **Title** Prompts to encourage appointment attendance for people with severe mental illness **Review type** Cochrane protocol **Objectives** To estimate the effects of simple prompting by professional carers to encourage compliance with care programmes for those with serious mental illness	**Search strategy** Biological Abstracts (1985 to 1999), CINAHL (1982 to 1999), Cochrane Schizophrenia Group's Register, Cochrane Library, EMBASE (1980 to 1999), MEDLINE (1966 to 1999), PsycLIT (1987 to September 1999) will all be searched for trials. In addition, ISI database- Science Citation Index, Social Science Citation Index and reference lists will be searched. The authors of all the studies initially selected for inclusion will be contacted. Finally, two journals will be handsearched. **Quality assessment** Reviewers will allocate trials to three quality categories, as described in the Cochrane Collaboration Handbook. Only trials in Category A or B will be included. **Statistical analysis** The reviewers will analyse data on an intention-to-treat basis where possible. For binary outcomes relative risk (RR) and 95% CI will be calculated, using a random effects model. **Quality score (assessed by reviewers):** N/a	**Types of studies** RCTs **Number of studies included** N/a **Years of studies:** N/a **Countries where studies undertaken** N/a	Anyone having been diagnosed with, or suspected of, a serious mental illness such as schizophrenia or schizophrenia-like illnesses, diagnosed by any criteria	In addition to standard care, any prompt or combination of prompts, whether text-based, electronic, by telephone call, personal visit, financial or other rewards that have the stated purpose of encouraging attendance. The comparison was standard care (not defined).	1. Service utilisation 2. Compliance: Other outcomes examined were classified under seven categories. 1. Death (suicides, all causes) 2. Service utilisation 3. Social functioning 4. Mental state 5. Quality of life 6. Satisfaction 7. Costs	N/a	N/a

*Cochrane reviews only

Review	Review Methodology	Included trial details	Participants	Intervention details	Outcomes	Results	Author's conclusions
Author Scott et al[29] **Date published (date last updated)*** 1995 **Title** Assertive community treatment and case management for schizophrenia **Review type** non-Cochrane **Objectives** To examine the impact of assertive community treatment (ACT) and case management models	**Search strategy** MEDLINE and PsycLIT were searched from 1966-1993 **Quality assessment** Data on research design, and sample criteria were collected **Statistical analysis** Narrative summary **Quality score (assessed by reviewers): 4**	**Types of studies** Reviews and RCTs **Number of studies included** 7 reviews and 12 RCTs with a total of 1,789 participants **Years of studies:** 1973-1995 **Countries where studies undertaken** Not stated	People with schizophrenia or severe mental illness	ACT as described by Stein and Test (1980) and ACT-like intensive case management was included with case management	Use of inpatient hospitalisation and community mental health services, costs and clinical and social outcome	ACT programmes reduce hospitalisation and increase use of community mental health services at an equivalent or reduced costs. Greater fidelity to the ACT model produced better outcomes. The impact of case management is less consistent, but intensive case management programmes also reduced hospitalisation.	ACT consistently reduces the rate and duration of psychiatric inpatient care, increases programme retention and may be less costly over the short- and mid-range compared with other methods of service delivery (e.g. community mental health centres or hospital-based aftercare). Intensive case management can also reduce inpatient utilisation and increase the rate of community-based services.

*Cochrane reviews only

Review	Author	Review Methodology	Included trial details	Participants	Intervention details	Outcomes	Results	Author's conclusions
Author Tyrer et al[24] **Date published (date last updated)*** 2000 (August 1998) **Title** Community mental health teams (CMHTs) for people with severe mental illnesses and disordered personality **Review type** Cochrane review **Objectives** To evaluate the effects of community mental health team (CMHT) treatment for anyone with serious mental illness		**Search strategy** Biological Abstracts (1982-1997), the Cochrane Library (1998, Issue 2), EMBASE (1980-1997), MEDLINE (1966-1997), PsycLIT (1974-1997) and SCISEARCH (1997) were searched for relevant trials. The Journal of Personality Disorders was hand searched, and contact was made with colleagues at ENMESH, ISSPD and in forensic psychiatry. **Quality assessment** Two reviewers independently rated the quality of all included studies using the Jadad Scale. Only trials reliably rating over 2 on this scale were included. **Statistical analysis** Where possible OR were calculated and an intention-to-treat analysis was undertaken. Tests of heterogeneity were undertaken. **Quality score (assessed by reviewers): 6**	**Types of studies** RCTs or quasi-RCTs **Number of studies included** Five RCTs with a total of 869 participants **Years of studies:** 1979-1998 **Countries where studies undertaken** UK: 3 Australia: 1 Canada: 1	Any individual presenting to, or being referred to, adult psychiatric services with severe mental illness (however diagnosed)	Community Mental Health Team: management of care from a multi disciplinary, community-based team The comparison was standard or usual care which must have been stated to be the normal care in the area concerned. Where this management was 'confounded' by a specific intervention, such as case-management or a team strategy (for example, Assertive Community Team management (ACT)), studies were excluded. However, if both groups, CMHT and 'standard care', received the specific intervention, then the study was appropriate to include.	The primary outcomes of interest were: death; violence; acceptability of management as measured by loss to follow up; and general improvement. Other outcomes were: hospitalisation; symptoms of serious mental illness; quality of life; participant and carer satisfaction; social functioning; economic costs of all care and health care	CMHT management may be associated with fewer deaths by suicide and in suspicious circumstances (OR 0.32, 95% CI: 0.09,1.12). It causes less people to be dissatisfied with their care (OR 0.34, 95% CI: 0.2-0.59) and to leave the studies early (OR 0.61, 95% CI: 0.45-0.83). No clear difference was found in admission rates, overall clinical outcomes and duration of in-patient hospital treatment, although this was partly a consequence of poorly presented data.	Community mental health team management is not inferior to non-team standard care in any important respects and is superior in promoting greater acceptance of treatment. It may also be superior in reducing hospital admission and avoiding death by suicide.

*Cochrane reviews only

Review	Review Methodology	Included trial details	Participants	Intervention details	Outcomes	Results	Author's conclusions
Author Wadhwa and Lavizzo-Mourey 28 **Date published (date last updated)*** 1999 **Title** Do innovative models of health care delivery improve quality of care for selected vulnerable populations? a systematic review **Review type** non-Cochrane **Objectives** To determine whether multidisciplinary teams, outreach or home care, and case management improve the quality of the care in two vulnerable populations - the terminally ill and the mentally ill	**Search strategy** MEDLINE (1977 to 1997), GENMED (1977 to 1997) were searched for articles in the English language. Manual searches of references from articles located through the computer search were also examined. Experts were contacted and authors of several articles were contacted to identify studies not found through the database. **Quality assessment** Data on the rigour of the studies were assessed including study conduct and analysis, including the reporting of an a priori sample size calculation, description of the randomisation process and adequacy of the follow-up period. Evidence was graded of the US Preventive Service Task Force quality of evidence. **Statistical analysis** Narrative summary **Quality score (assessed by reviewers):** 5	**Types of studies** Controlled studies **Number of studies included** 14 RCTs with a total of 2,161 participants **Years of studies:** 1979-1994 **Countries where studies undertaken** UK: 6 USA: 4 Australia: 1 Unknown: 3	People with a severe mental illness	A combination of one or more of the three models of innovative care: multidisciplinary teams, home care and case management. Comparison was conventional care.	Quality of care, defined as the 'degree to which health services for individuals and populations increase the likelihood of desired health outcomes and are consistent with current professional knowledge.' Outcomes included in the studies were assessment of utilisation, satisfaction, costs and symptoms.	Multidisciplinary outreach strategies were effective in reducing inpatient hospitalisations. Costs were inadequately assessed in the studies to draw a summary conclusion.	Multidisciplinary outreach programmes for the mentally ill resulted in lower inpatient utilisation and similar clinical outcomes, including reduced severity of symptoms and a more rapid and larger improvement in functioning at all costs. Aggressive case management strategies were beneficial for the mentally ill, although the cost were not assessed.

*Cochrane reviews only

Review	Review Methodology	Included trial details	Participants	Intervention details	Outcomes	Results	Author's conclusions
Author Wing et al[38] **Date published (date last updated)*** 1998 **Title** Management of imminent violence: clinical practice guidelines to support mental health services **Review type** non-Cochrane **Objectives** To determine whether there was a base of solid research evidence on which clinical guidelines could be founded	**Search strategy** MEDLINE (1966-1997), EMBASE (1986 to 1996), PsycLIT (1974 to 1997) and the Cochrane Library (1997: issue 3) were searched for relevant trials. Also, review articles were scanned for additional references and a range of experts were contacted. **Quality assessment** Consideration was given to clarity of hypotheses, size and adequacy of sampling procedures, drop-out rates, the appropriate use of measurement tools and statistical analyses and a clear disinterested presentation. **Statistical analysis** Narrative summary **Quality score (assessed by reviewers):** 5	**Types of studies** All types of studies **Number of studies included** 68 studies were included, but only those evaluating the prediction of imminent violence were relative to this review (16 trials of which 13 were cohort and three were descriptive). **Years of studies:** 1983-1996 **Countries where studies undertaken** Not stated	People in mental health care settings who are violent or where violence is imminent	Interventions which, in acute clinical settings, predict with reasonable accuracy which patients are most likely to become aggressive or violent in the near future	Accuracy in the prediction assessment of violence	The studies do not provide a clear consensus on items that would be clinically useful for short-term prediction. This does not mean that prediction (still less assessment) is impossible; only that no generalisation can be made from these results.	Considered in the context of the other subjects, it would seem useful to include in the list of terms to be considered variables such as quality of environment and training and interventions such as one-to-one observation ('specialising') and medication, which aim to influence outcome in the short term.

*Cochrane reviews only

NSF standard six: caring about carers

Review	Review Methodology	Included trial details	Participants	Intervention details	Outcomes	Results	Author's conclusions
Author Cuijpers[51] **Date published (date last updated)*** 1999 **Title** The effects of family interventions on relatives' burden: a meta-analysis **Review type** non-Cochrane **Objectives** To test the hypothesis that family interventions have a positive effect on the burden of relatives of psychiatric patients	**Search strategy** PsycLIT and MEDLINE were searched from 1966 to 1993 **Quality assessment** Data were collected on use of a control group, random assignment to condition, data on drop-out, follow-up measurements, use of reliable measure and reported in a table **Statistical analysis** Effect sizes were calculated for each study and then combined into a summary effect size **Quality score (assessed by reviewers): 4**	**Types of studies** RCTs, controlled trials or pre-post test studies **Number of studies included** 16 studies (9 RCTs, 5 non-RCTs) and two pre-test post test studies (total number of participants not stated) **Years of studies:** 1987-1996 **Countries where studies undertaken** Not stated	Relatives of psychiatric patients	Family interventions. These ranged from one educational session to intensive family treatment. Many interventions included information, discussion, sharing and coping strategies.	A measure that could be classified as an element of the relatives' burden of care. 1. Relatives' psychological distress 2. Relationship with patient (e.g. feelings and attitudes) 3. Family functioning (e.g. conflict, sense of disruption, satisfaction)	An analysis of the 16 studies that were found, indicate that family interventions can have considerable effects on relatives' burden, psychological distress, the relationship between patient and relative and family functioning. Large effects are found in a subset of six studies. Interventions with more than 12 sessions have larger effects than shorter interventions. Several other success predictors can be hypothesised to be related to outcome.	Family interventions for relatives of psychiatric patients can have considerable effects on relatives' burden. Family interventions can have considerable effects on the relatives' psychological distress, the relationship between the patient and the relative, and family functioning. However, intervention with less than ten sessions have no important effects on relatives' burden.

*Cochrane reviews only

Review	Review Methodology	Included trial details	Participants	Intervention details	Outcomes	Results	Author's conclusions
Author Flint [52] **Date published (date last updated)*** 1995 **Title** Effects of respite care on patients with dementia and their caregivers **Review type** non-Cochrane **Objectives** To determine the effect of formal respite care on patients with dementia and their caregivers	**Search strategy** MEDLINE, PsycINFO, and CINAHL were searched from 1975 to 1994 for English language articles. Bibliographies of retrieved articles were searched for additional references. **Quality assessment** Validity was assessed on the following criteria: treatment and control groups were randomised or had baseline comparability, all patients entering the study were accounted for in its conclusions and statistical and clinical significance were considered. **Statistical analysis** Narrative summary **Quality score (assessed by reviewers):** 4	**Types of studies** Controlled trials **Number of studies included** 4 controlled trials were included with a total of 762 participants **Years of studies:** 1988-1992 **Countries where studies undertaken** Not stated	People with dementia who were living at home and their caregivers. No standardised criteria were used to make the diagnosis of dementia.	Respite care which was defined as a care giving service that provided a planned, temporary break from the ongoing responsibility of caring for a person with dementia who is living at home. Forms of respite care studied included institution, in-home and day-care. The duration of respite care ranged from 15 days to 12 months.	Outcome measures selected included those that assessed the caregivers burden and stress, psychiatric status, physical health and attitudes toward the patient, those that assessed the dementia patient's cognition, behaviour, physical health and functioning and the length of time the patient remains in the community.	Factors limiting the reliability of the results include: lack of standardised criteria to make the diagnosis of dementia, use of more than one type of respite care intervention with pooling of results, no controlling for contamination, use of respite service out with the study by control groups, additional counselling being given to treatment groups receiving respite care and groups already receiving formal community services at the time of entry. Caregiver: Burden and stress no difference; psychiatric status no difference; physical health no difference; attitude toward patient worse post respite (P <0.01).	Based on the results of controlled studies there is little evidence that respite care for a patient with dementia significantly affects caregiver burden or delays institutionalisation of the patient. However, given the small number of studies and methodological and conceptual problems these data are far from conclusive and benefits of respite care might be demonstrated in the future through better designed trials.

*Cochrane reviews only

Review	Review Methodology	Included trial details	Participants	Intervention details	Outcomes	Results	Author's conclusions
Author McNally et al[53] **Date published (date last updated)*** 1999 **Title** The effects of respite care on informal carers' well-being: a systematic review **Review type** non-Cochrane **Objectives** To examine research on respite provision with a view to establishing what effect it has on carers	**Search strategy** PsycLIT (1974-1997), MEDLINE(1966-1997), and the Social Science Citation Index (1996-1997) were searched for relevant trials **Quality assessment** Not stated, but discussed methodological issues **Statistical analysis** Narrative summary **Quality score (assessed by reviewers): 4**	**Types of studies** RCTs, quasi-experimental studies, and uncontrolled studies **Number of studies included** Five RCTs, 6 quasi-experimental, 1 study using a single-case study comparison and 17 uncontrolled studies (2865 participants in total) **Years of studies:** 1985-1995 **Countries where studies undertaken** Not stated	Informal carers of people with a range of physical and medical problems. Ten of the studies were of carers of people suffering from Alzheimer's or dementia	Respite care - four main categories: 'inpatient' residential respite care, out of home 'day care, out of home 'overnight' care and 'in home' respite (which usually involved scheduled visits from a nurse/care assistant)	Carers' well-being. Specific outcomes included in the studies were psychological well-being, carer stress or carer burden, and physical health	There was little evidence that respite intervention has either a consistent or enduring beneficial effect on carers' well-being. This may be due in part to the fact that the majority of the work conducted has been methodologically poor. Also significant, however, may be that the findings suggest respite care often fails to facilitate the maintenance of socially supportive relationships, which may moderate strain after respite has ended.	A more 'carer-centred' approach is required in both the provision and evaluation of respite care intervention. This approach would address the experience of both caregiver and care-recipient during the respite period.

*Cochrane reviews only

Review	Included trial details	Review Methodology	Participants	Intervention details	Outcomes	Results	Author's conclusions
Author Thompson and Briggs[54] **Date published (date last updated)*** May 1998 **Title** Support for carers of people with Alzheimer's type dementia **Review type** Cochrane review **Objectives** To provide an assessment of the effectiveness of health and/or social interventions designed to help support the carers of people with Alzheimer's-type dementias	**Types of studies** RCTs **Number of studies included** Six RCTs with over 301 participants (numbers not given for one study) **Years of studies:** 1989-1995 **Countries where studies undertaken** All undertaken in the USA or Canada	**Search strategy** The Cochrane Controlled Trials Register was searched for relevant trials. **Quality assessment** The two reviewers independently assigned each selected study to quality categories described in the Cochrane Collaboration Handbook and the NHS Centre for Reviews and Dissemination. Other elements of study quality which were noted were: i) 'blinding' of either service providers or service recipients to the nature of their allocated grouping ii) the level of carer drop-out at the follow-up stage iii) any follow up analysis of those leaving the study iv) equal treatment of both intervention and control groups **Statistical analysis** Narrative summary. Due to heterogeneity, a qualitative overview was deemed the most appropriate strategy. **Quality score (assessed by reviewers):** 5	Informal carers of people diagnosed as having dementia of the Alzheimer's type (an informal carer is defined as a person providing care, free of charge, to an individual with dementia in a home or non-institutional environment)	The interventions reviewed are those commonly provided by health and/or social services. These may or may not involve temporarily removing the person being cared for from the caring environment. The interventions were classified as: specialised respite services individualised service assessment and planning technology-based networking (e.g. computer bulletin boards and specialist telephone networks) carer education/training multi-faceted/dimensional strategies (i.e. those which utilise more than one approach; for example, specialist assessment and training).	Carer's quality of life and/or physical health as measured by validated indicators. Data on health or social services use such as numbers of health/social services contacts, numbers of resources used and frequency. Carer's mental health as measured by psychiatric morbidity indicators Financial cost data.	The results of the review are inconclusive. No evidence was found for the following comparison interventions: 1) individualised service assessment and planning versus conventional support; 2) technology-based carer networking (via computers or telephones) versus conventional support; 3) carer-education/training versus conventional support; 4) multi-faceted/dimensional strategies (such as specialised carer assessment and training) versus conventional support.	With the limited nature of the research evidence in mind, it is not possible to recommend either wholesale investment in caregiver support programmes or withdrawal of the same. With the addition of further studies in future updates of this review, expected in early 1999, this presently inconclusive picture may become clearer.

*Cochrane reviews only

NSF standard seven: preventing suicide

Review	Included trial details	Review Methodology	Participants	Intervention details	Outcomes	Results	Author's conclusions
Author Hawton et al **Date published (date last updated)*** 1999 **Title** Psychosocial versus pharmacological treatments for deliberate self-harm **Review type** Cochrane review and published review **Objectives** To synthesise the findings from RCTs that have examined effectiveness of treatments of patients who have deliberately harmed themselves	**Types of studies** RCTs **Number of studies included** 23 RCTs with a total of 3014 participants **Years of studies:** 1973-1999 **Countries where studies undertaken** UK: 13 USA/Canada: 4 Ireland: 1 Europe: 5	**Search strategy** MEDLINE (1966-1999), PsycLIT (1974-1999) Embase (1980-1999); The Cochrane Controlled Trials Register (CCTR) No.1 1999. Ten journals in the field of psychiatry and psychology were hand searched for the first version of this review. Reference lists of papers were checked and trialists contacted. **Quality assessment** The quality of the papers was rated by two independent reviewers blind to their authorship according to the recommended Cochrane criteria for quality assessment. **Statistical analysis** Summary odds ratios were calculated **Quality score (assessed by reviewers):** 7	Males and females of all ages, who shortly before entering the study had all engaged in any type of deliberately initiated self-poisoning or self-harm. Trials in which the participants were suicide ideators (without self-harm) or those of people with depression in which deliberate self-harm was an outcome variable were not included.	All psychosocial and/or psychopharmacological treatment. Studies were grouped as: 1. problem solving therapy vs. standard aftercare 2. intensive intervention plus outreach (e.g. home-based treatment either as standard or for those patients who defaulted on appointments at a clinic). 3. emergency card vs. standard after care - included studies in which experimental group were given an emergency contact card with which they either had 24-hour access to emergency advice from a psychiatrist, or could admit themselves to hospital. In only one other group 4. Antidepressant medication vs. placebo	The main outcome measure was the rate of repeated self-harm (fatal and non-fatal) within a follow-up period of up to 2 years. Other outcomes included compliance with treatment, depression, hopelessness, suicidal ideation/thoughts, change in problems/problem resolution.	The summary OR indicated a trend towards reduced repetition of deliberate self-harm for problem-solving therapy compared with standard aftercare (OR 0.70, 95% CI: 0.45 to 1.11) and for provision of an emergency contact card in addition to standard care compared with standard aftercare alone (0.45, 95% CI: 0.19 to 1.07). The summary OR for trials of intensive aftercare plus outreach compared with standard aftercare was 0.83 (95% CI:0.61 to 1.14), and for antidepressant treatment compared with placebo was 0.83 (95% CI:0.47 to 1.48). The remainder of the comparisons were in single small trials.	There still remains considerable uncertainty about which forms of psychosocial and physical treatments of self-harm patients are most effective, insufficient numbers of patients in trials being the main limiting factor. There is a need for larger trials of treatments associated with trends towards reduced rates of repetition of deliberate self-harm. The results of small single trials which have been associated with statistically significant reductions in repetition must be interpreted with caution and it is desirable that such trials are also replicated.

*Cochrane reviews only

Review	Review Methodology	Included trial details	Participants	Intervention details	Outcomes	Results	Author's conclusions
Author Johnson et al[55] **Date published (date last updated)*** 1999 **Title** The role of objective personality inventories in suicide risk assessment: An evaluation and proposal **Review type** non-Cochrane **Objectives** To review the empirical literature regarding the efficacy of established personality inventories in preventing suicide	**Search strategy** PsycLIT (Jan 1974-March 1996) was searched for relevant trials. Foreign language trials were excluded. Reference lists were searched for additional trials. **Quality assessment** None stated **Statistical analysis** Narrative summary **Quality score (assessed by reviewers):** 3	**Types of studies** Trials used one of the risk assessment measure in its entirety and compared it with one or more subscale in isolation **Number of studies included** 42 (number of participants not stated) **Years of studies:** 1975-1994 **Countries where studies undertaken** Not stated	Subjects with a clear history of suicide ideation and/or attempts, subjects with current suicide ideation, or subjects having made a recent suicide gesture or attempt. Psychotic patients were excluded.	Objective personality assessment instruments including California Personality Inventory; Edwards Preference Schedule; Eysenck Personality Tests; Millon Clinical Multiaxial Inventory (I-III); Minnesota Multiphasic Personality Inventory (1-2) ; Myers-Briggs Type Indicator; 16 Personality Factor Test; Neuroticism, Extroversion, Openness Personality Inventory; Personality Diagnostic Questionnaire	Prediction of suicidal intention	There was scant evidence for most of the scales. Even for the most frequently utilised and researched inventory, the Minnesota Multiphasic Personality Inventory (MMPI), no single scale or configural profile has proven consistently predictive of suicidal behaviour. The only exception appears to be that elevated scores on the Mf (Masculinity-femininity) scale show some consistency in relation to suicidality. The MMPI has generally not proven consistently useful in discriminating either suicide attempters or ideators from nonsuicidal persons.	Unifying themes on the scanty research on personality inventories in suicide assessment included marked heterogeneity in research design quality and lack of evidence for predictive utility on the part of the inventories reviews. The review highlights a wide range of methodological shortcomings in this research and very little evidence of consistent predictive utility for any single inventory, scale or item.

*Cochrane reviews only

Review	Review Methodology	Included trial details	Participants	Intervention details	Outcomes	Results	Author's conclusions
Author Repper[57] **Date published (date last updated)*** 1999 **Title** A review of the literature on the prevention of suicide through interventions in accident and emergency departments **Review type** non-Cochrane **Objectives** To identify the most effective adult suicide prevention interventions in A&E departments	**Search strategy** MEDLINE CINAHL, and the Science Citation Index were searched to identify relevant English language papers reporting studies/review undertaken since 1990. Reference lists were also searched. **Quality assessment** Not stated **Statistical analysis** Narrative summary, clear results not presented **Quality score (assessed by reviewers): 3**	**Types of studies** All types of studies **Number of studies included** 7 RCTs to reduce deliberate self-harm with a total of 1,290 participants **Years of studies:** 1973-1990 **Countries where studies undertaken** Not stated	People with a history of deliberate self-harm (e.g. self-poisoning) or at risk of suicide.	Interventions included psychiatric appointments, social work task-centred work; home versus outpatient treatment; counselling; inpatient vs outpatient psychotherapy; cognitive-behavioural therapy.	Reduction in deliberate self-harm and reduction in the risk of suicide	No suicide prevention strategies have been conclusively demonstrated to be effective. Three distinct groups of A&E attendees at particular risk of suicide were identified: 1. Deliberate self-harm; 2. People with specific physical problems; 3. People with a history of mental health problems.	Action to reduce suicide needs to be taken at all levels of the organisation. The role of the suicide prevention nurse needs to include support, training and development. It should also include specific time limited therapy with a highly targeted group of patients at specific risk.

*Cochrane reviews only

Review	Review Methodology	Included trial details	Participants	Intervention details	Outcomes	Results	Author's conclusions
Author Van der Sande et al[58] **Date published (date last updated)*** 1997 **Title** Psychosocial intervention following suicide attempt: a systematic review of treatment interventions **Review type** non-Cochrane **Objectives** To assess the effectiveness of interventions for suicide attempters by a systematic review of RCTs	**Search strategy** MEDLINE (1966-December 1995), PsycLIT (1974 to December 1995) were searched for relevant trials. English language literature only was included. **Quality assessment** Information on methodological aspects of the studies were reported and used when assessing the strength of evidence provided by the review. In particular, method of ascertainment and use of intention to treat analyses were reported. **Statistical analysis** Random-effects meta-analysis **Quality score (assessed by reviewers):** 6	**Types of studies** RCTs **Number of studies included** 15 RCTs (total of 2019 participants). Psychiatric management of poor compliance with aftercare: 6 studies found (n= 1023 patients). Guaranteed in-patient shelter: 2 studies (n= 317 patients). Psychosocial crisis intervention: 2 studies (n= 480 patients). Cognitive-behavioural treatment: 4 studies (n= 122 patients). **Years of studies:** check **Countries where studies undertaken** Not known	Suicide attempters. Attempted suicide was defined as including deliberate self-poisoning and deliberate self-harm. Studies on mentally handicapped people, or people with learning disabilities were excluded. The trials included with a range of psychiatric morbidities, including depression, alcohol/drug and substance use, neurosis, personality disorder, reactive disorder, mood disorder, anxiety disorder, depressive disorder, psychiatric disturbance, GHQ positive cases, and dysthymia.	Psychosocial/psychotherapeutic interventions. These were grouped into 4 categories: psychiatric management of poor compliance with aftercare, guaranteed in-patient shelter, psychosocial crisis intervention, and cognitive-behavioural treatment.	The primary outcome was the incidence of repeated suicide attempts	Psychiatric management of poor compliance with aftercare: summary RR=0.81 (95% CI:0.6,1.2), based on 5 homogenous studies out of 6 (1 was excluded as it contributed to heterogeneity). Guaranteed in-patient shelter: Based on 2 studies, no significant reduction in RR (summary RR= 0.5, 95% CI:0.2,1.1). Psychosocial crisis intervention: Based on 2 studies, summary RR=0.9 (95%CI:0.5,1.3). Cognitive-behavioural treatment: Based on 4 studies, summary RR=0.5 (95%CI:0.3, 0.8).	No clear evidence was found for a reduction in repeated suicide attempts with interventions which seek to increase compliance with aftercare, or which guarantee in-patient shelter in the event of an emergency or psychosocial crisis. Only cognitive-behavioural therapy appeared to significantly reduce the incidence of repeated suicide attempts. However, some aspects of the available trials on this intervention leave room for uncertainty about the magnitude of effect the extent to which the results may be extrapolated to other subgroups.

*Cochrane reviews only

APPENDIX 4. SCOPING 24-HOUR MENTAL HEALTH SERVICES

Zelda Di Blasi, Kath Wright, Ruth Jepson, Gerben Ter Riet
Date prepared and circulated: 02 July 2000

INTRODUCTION

The need for twenty-four hour mental health services has been highlighted by individuals with mental illness and their carers[90] and by various governmental documents. More recently the National Service Framework on Mental Health[1] emphasised that all people with mental health problems should be able to access local services round the clock, 365 days a year. They should also be able to use NHS direct for first-level advice and referral to specialist helplines or to local services. What is not clear is the extent to which these services are actually effective and cost-effective models of care.

The NHS Centre for Reviews and Dissemination was asked by the Department of Health to systematically review the evidence for the effectiveness of 24-hour and out-of-hours mental health services. The present document aims to explore the feasibility of conducting such a review, by scoping the topic to identify current thinking, gain an estimation of the size of the literature and facilitate question refinement.

24-hour and out-of-hours mental health services

There appear to be two main types of 24-hour services: 'crisis' and 'planned' out-of-hour services.[90] *Crisis services* are urgent responses from mental health services for people with severe mental illnesses. In 1995 MIND[91] identified 24-hour crisis services as having seven components:

- a crisis helpline;
- a crisis counselling service;
- crisis houses;
- crisis beds in the community;
- home treatment service;
- after-hours phone link to teams/workers; and
- acute in-patient services.

Planned 24-hour services aim to anticipate, pre-empt, contain or avoid crises. These services are less defined and less researched than crisis services. Examples are drop-in clubhouses and community group networks, which provide social support, leisure or activities that aim to enhance employment prospects.

As part of a scoping review of mental health service delivery, the present authors identified various reviews that are likely to contain some aspect of 24-hour care. These have been tabulated in (see table). Community or home treatment services seem to be the most extensively researched types of crisis services.

LITERATURE SEARCHES

Specific literature searches were conducted to identify studies that focused on out-of-hours or 24-hours services. From some initial exploration undertaken to identify relevant studies for this review a number of difficulties in conducting a reliable literature search were identified. Following this initial search, two strategies (A and B) were developed to try and overcome some of the problems.

Strategy A
Version 1
The first MEDLINE (1966-2000) strategy produced contained the following sets:
set a mental health services
set b mental health
set c 24 hour services
set d emergency psych/crisis management

set e   helplines
set f   day care

These were combined as follows:
set a or set c or set d or set e or set f (set b was used to limit the results of sets d,e and f)

This MEDLINE search retrieved a total of 39,640 records. Unique records are also expected to be identified in both PsycLIT and EMBASE. It will be difficult to focus the search strategy more clearly without being very specific as to the models of service provision the review is considering.

Version 2
To restrict the search, terms associated to 24-hour services ('7 days a week', round the clock' etc.) were combined with 'mental health' and 'mental health services'.

set a   24 hour services,
set b   7 days a week,
set c   round the clock,
set d   on call services,
set e   out of hours services,
set f   after hours services.
set g   mental health
set h   mental health services

This search resulted in 308 hits. Of these, 44 records appeared to be relevant. The majority of these articles were case studies of telephone services and alternatives to hospital accommodation or epidemiological studies attempting to identify high 24-hour service users. With the exception of one study, all the clinical trials identified in this search were related to home-based crisis services, which are well covered by systematic reviews.

The terms regularly used to refer to the provision of services (24 hour services, 7 days a week, round the clock, on call services, out of hours services, after hours services) can only be used as search terms in databases in the following format: 24-hour services, out-of-hour, after-hour, drop-in etc. It is not possible to search for words such as "out", "after'" etc. as individual search terms because database providers designate such common words as "stop-words". It is not clear how reliable searching for phrases such as "after-hours" is, but there is some cause for uncertainty as the initial scoping search of MEDLINE retrieved a total of 39,640 records but only 308 of this number contained one of these terms.

Version 3
In this version, the strategy was re-organised to create the following sets:
set a   mental health (used to limit sets c,d,e)
set b   24 hrs
set c   emergency psych.
set d   helplines
set e   day care

This search resulted in 18,056 records. This is still possibly an unmanageable number of records especially as this did not include the MESH headings community mental health services, mental health services, social work psychiatric, psychiatric nursing. Although this set of terms seem to be appropriate, these studies should be combined with appropriate terms.

Version 4
The scope of 'set a' was widened to include mental health services as well as mental health.
set a   mental health or mental health services
set b   24 hrs etc
set c   emergency psych.
set d   helplines
set e   day care

In this version 'set a' has been used to limit all of the other sets and the sets are combined as follows: set b or set c or set d or set e. This approach retrieves 13,000 records approx. Although this is a more manageable number this search may potentially miss relevant studies.

Strategy B
One way of checking a strategy is to see whether a number of known studies are identified by it. In a report of out-of-hours services, Jones reviewed 12 studies evaluating interventions that incorporated a 24-hour crisis response.[90] Of these studies, 10 are on MEDLINE, but only 6 of them are retrieved by the search strategy, version 4. Furthermore, of the 10 MEDLINE studies referred to above, only two specifically refer to 24 hours or out of hours.

RECOMMENDATIONS
As can be gathered from the literature searches described in this document, the main difficulty in evaluating the effectiveness of 24-hour mental health services relates to the definition of the '24-hour' or 'out-of-hours' concept. Since there is a wide range of services that are providing 24-hour services by definition, there is a strong possibility that they won't actually mention the provision of out-of-hours services, as this will just be implied. The term 24-hours is therefore not applicable to a comprehensive and thorough review of these services. It would be more useful to identify studies of specific mental health service delivery which are likely to incorporate 24-hour care.

The present authors identified various reviews of such studies as part of a scoping review. These studies have been tabulated in the appendix. Two areas identified by this review as not being covered by systematic reviews were round-the-clock contact with local services and telephone helplines. It is possible that empirical research evaluating the effectiveness of these services has not been conducted to date. A review in these areas would therefore cover a gap in the literature, possibly recommending that primary research be carried out to evaluate the effectiveness and cost-effectiveness of these interventions.

In deciding which studies to review, it is necessary to prioritise, focus research questions and establish appropriate comparisons. In doing so, it is important to evaluate specific types of services. These may be single component (e.g. helplines) or multi-component (e.g. assertive outreach, crisis intervention). In this case, it would be necessary to decide whether to evaluate the components of 24-hours services (e.g. to establish whether a 24 hour helpline is more effective than a daytime helpline) or the methods of gaining access to the services (e.g. to estimate the (cost-)effectiveness of a telephone helpline in making 24-hour services accessible to people).

CONCLUSION
For purposes of systematic reviewing the concept of 24-hour care is not useful. A number of good reviews on the effectiveness of specific services that provide 24-hour care exist. Further reviews of other specific services that provide 24-hour care may be considered after prudent prioritisation.

SYSTEMATIC REVIEWS WHICH ARE LIKELY TO CONTAIN SOME ASPECT OF 24-HOUR CARE

Review	Types of studies/years	Participants	Intervention details	Primary outcomes
Community or home based care interventions				
Holloway et al, 1995[26] Non-Cochrane review	RCTs, matched-control, repeated measures (own-control), and descriptive studies	People with psychiatric disorder or disability	Brokerage case management and clinical case management	Number of hospital days and admissions, costs, use of community care services, satisfaction with services, quality of life, symptoms, social functioning
Marshall et al, 1997*[2] Cochrane review	RCTs	People with a severe mental illness	Case management (UK terms 'care management' and 'care program approach')	Numbers remaining in contact with psychiatric services, extent of psychiatric hospital admissions, clinical, social outcomes, and costs
Mueser et al, 1998[27] Non-Cochrane review	RCTs, controlled and non-controlled studies	People with a severe mental illness	Standard case management (broker and clinical case management), ACT, intensive case management, strengths case management, rehabilitation case management	Time in hospital, symptoms, social adjustment, housing stability, jail/arrests, substance abuse, medication compliance, quality of life, vocational functioning, patient and relative satisfaction
Wadhwa and Lavizzo-Mourey, 1999[28] Non-Cochrane review	Controlled studies	People with a severe mental illness	Multidisciplinary teams, home care and case management	Quality of care
Joy et al, 2000*[34] Cochrane review	RCTs	People with a severe mental illness	Crisis intervention	Hospitalisation, patient, carer and staff satisfaction with treatment, clinical outcomes
Latimer, 1999[31] Non-Cochrane review	RCTs, pre-post studies and controlled studies	People with a severe mental illness	Assertive community treatment	Time spent in hospital
Marshall & Lockwood, 1998*[30] Cochrane review	RCTs	People with a severe mental illness	Assertive community treatment, assertive case management or 'PACT'	Remaining in contact with the psychiatric services, extent of psychiatric hospital admissions, clinical and social outcome and costs
Scott et al, 1995[29] Non-Cochrane review	Reviews and RCTs	People with a severe mental illness	ACT as described by Stein and Test (1980)	Use of inpatient hospitalisation and community mental health services, costs and clinical and social outcome
Burns et al, Ongoing Unpublished review	Controlled trials	People with a severe mental illness	Community or home based care interventions that do not readily fall within case management, ACT or crisis Intervention	
Tyrer et al, 1998*[24] Cochrane review	RCTs or quasi-RCTs	People with a severe mental illness	Community Mental Health Teams	Death, violence, acceptability of management as measured by loss to follow up, and general improvement
Systematic reviews to improve the organisation of primary care				
Abi-Aad et al, 2000 (expected end 2001)[17] Cochrane protocol	RCTs, controlled before and after studies (CBA), and interrupted time series studies (ITS)	Patients with minor illness or injury attending hospital emergency departments	Interventions in which primary or community care professionals provide care for new attenders at the hospital A&E department	Service use including diagnostic interventions, treatments, referrals to specialist care, hospital admission

Review	Types of studies/years	Participants	Intervention details	Primary outcomes
Supported employment and vocational rehabilitation				
Bond et al, 1997[44] Non-Cochrane review	Pre-post studies, surveys, quasi-RCTs and non-RCTs	People with a severe mental illness	Vocational programmes offering supported employment	Employment rate
Crowther et al, 1999 (expected mid-2000)[46] Cochrane protocol	RCTs	People with a severe mental illness	Vocational rehabilitation	Number of people in competitive employment at the end of the study
Lehman, 1995[45] Non-Cochrane review	Controlled trials	People with a severe mental illness	Vocational rehabilitation, sheltered workshops, rehabilitation counselling, assertive community treatment and job developer	Vocational functioning
Nicol et al, 1998*[47] Cochrane review	RCTs or quasi-RCTs	People with a severe mental illness	Life skills programmes	Self-care functioning at personal and domestic level (life skills)
Day care and day hospitals				
Almaraz-Serrano et al, 1997 (expected mid-2000)[48] Cochrane protocol	RCTs reporting data on an intention-to-treat basis	People with a severe mental illness	Day hospital care or day time attendance at a facility	Numbers maintaining contact with the services, extent of hospital care received, clinical and social outcomes, costs of care
Catty et al, 1999 (expected mid-2000)[37] Cochrane protocol	RCTs comparing day centres with standard care or day hospital care	People with a severe mental illness	Day centre care	Death, suicide or natural causes, leaving the study early, clinical response, violent or criminal behaviour, service use, economic outcomes, quality of life / satisfaction with care
Brooker et al, 1996[25] Non-Cochrane review - two papers	RCTs and quasi-RCTs	Individuals with mental health problems	Community mental health nursing interventions	Depression, anxiety, fear, general health, hopelessness, social adjustment and process measures
Supported housing				
Hayes and Macdonald, 1999[5] (expected mid-2000) Cochrane protocol	RCTs. Quasi-randomized trials will also be identified for a sensitivity analysis	People with a severe mental illness	Supported housing schemes or outreach support schemes	Service utilisation, medical/mental state changes, professional support workers' satisfaction and tenant or respondent satisfaction, social functioning, quality of life, economic outcomes

*For Cochrane reviews, date last updated

APPENDIX 5. SEARCH STRATEGY FOR IDENTIFYING ECONOMIC EVALUATIONS OF MENTAL HEALTH SERVICE DELIVERY INTERVENTIONS

A5.1 NHS EED

This database is produced and maintained by the NHS CRD. Economic evaluations were identified by searching the following databases regularly: Current Contents-Clinical Medicine (1994 onwards), MEDLINE (1995 onwards), CINAHL (1995 onwards). NHS EED includes records of economic evaluations, cost-benefit analyses, cost-utility analyses, and cost-effectiveness analyses. Cost-minimisation analyses and cost-consequence analyses were also included. The search will be carried out on the administrative version of the database.

The search strategy used will be:
1. mental
2. depress or schizophrenia
3. stress
4. eating(w)disorder
5. panic or phobia or anxiety
6. psychiatric or counselling or counseling
7. psychotherap$
8. psychiatrist$
9. 1 or 2 or 3 or 4 or 5 or 6 or 7 or 8
10. SAW/st1 and 9
11. SAC/st1 and 9
12. 10 or 11

Note: SAW indicates "structured abstract being written", SAC indicates "structured abstract on the public database"

A5.2 HMIC

This database (the Health Management Information Consortium) contains records from the Department of Health Library (1983-March 2000), the King's Fund Library (1979-March 2000) and HELMIS (1984-1998) from the University of Leeds. It is a useful database for identifying the grey literature.

The search strategy used will be:
- #1 cost effect*
- #2 cost util*
- #3 cost benefit
- #4 economic evaluation*
- #5 #1 or #2 or #3 or #4
- #6 mental* or depress* or schizophren*
- #7 stress or eating disorder*
- #8 bulimia or anorexia
- #9 panic or phobia* or anxiety
- #10 psychiatric or counselling or counseling
- #11 psychotherap*
- #12 psychiatrist*
- #13 #6 or #7 or #8 or #9 or #10 or #11 or #12
- #14 #5 and #13

A5.3 EMBASE

Embase (on Silverplatter) will be searched for the period 1985-March 2000 using the strategy below:

- #1 explode "mental-disease"/ all subheadings
- #2 explode "mental-health"/ all subheadings
- #3 "anxiety"/ all subheadings

#4	explode "mental-health-care"/ all subheadings
#5	explode "psychiatric-treatment"/ all subheadings
#6	explode "schizophrenia"/ all subheadings
#7	#1 or #2 or #3 or #4 or #5 or #6
#8	(explode "economic-evaluation"/ all subheadings) and #7
#9	"cost-benefit-analysis"/ all subheadings
#10	"cost-effectiveness-analysis"/ all subheadings
#11	"cost-minimization-analysis"/ all subheadings
#12	"cost-utility-analysis"/ all subheadings
#13	"economic-evaluation"/ all subheadings
#14	#9 or #10 or #11 or #12 or #13
#15	#7 and #14
#16	PY > "1985"
#17	#15 and (PY > "1985")

A5.4 PsycLIT

PsycLIT (on Silverplatter) will be searched for the period 1985-Dec 1999 using the strategy below:

#1	explode "Costs-and-Cost-Analysis"
#2	economic near (evaluation in ti)
#3	cost* near (benefit* in ti)
#4	cost* near (utilit* in ti)
#5	cost* near (effective* in ti)
#6	cost* near (stud* in ti)
#7	cost* near (minimi* in ti)
#8	cost* near (analys* in ti)
#9	program* near (cost* in ti)
#10	economic near (cost* in ti)
#11	cost* near (mental in ti)
#12	economic near (mental in ti)
#13	cost* near (psych* in ti)
#14	economic* near (psych* in ti)
#15	compara* near (economic* in ti)
#16	expenditure near (mental in ti)
#17	expenditure near (psych* in ti)
#18	cost near (efficien* in ti)
#19	#1 or #2 or #3 or #4 or #5 or #6 or #7 or #8 or #9 or #10 or #11 or #12 or #13 or #14 or #15 or #16 or #17 or #18 or #19

A5.5 MEDLINE

MEDLINE (on Silverplatter) will be searched for the period 1966-1993 using the strategy below. The search of NHS EED will have provided coverage of MEDLINE for the period 1994 to date.

The search strategy used will be:

#1	explode "costs-and-cost-analysis"/all subheadings in mjme
#2	economic near (evaluat* in ti)
#3	cost* near (benefit* in ti)
#4	cost* near (utilit* in ti)
#5	cost* near (effective* in ti)
#6	cost* near (stud* in ti)
#7	cost* near (minimi* in ti)
#8	cost* near (analys* in ti)
#9	program* near (cost* in ti)
#10	economic near (cost* in ti)
#11	cost* near (mental in ti)
#12	economic near (mental in ti)
#13	cost* near (psych* in ti)
#14	economic* near (psych* in ti)
#15	compara* near (economic* in ti)

#16	expenditure near (mental in ti)
#17	expenditure near (psych* in ti)
#18	cost near (efficien* in ti)
#19	#1 or #2 or #3 or #4 or #5 or #6 or #7 or #8 or #9 or #10 or #11 or #12 or #13 or #14 or #15 or #16 or #17 or #18 or #19
#20	"mental-health"/all subheadings
#21	explode "mental-health-services"/all subheadings
#22	explode "psychiatry"/all subheadings
#23	explode "mental-disorders"/all subheadings
#24	#20 or #21 or #22 or #23
#59	#19 and #24

A5.6 OHE HEED database

OHE HEED on CD ROM will be searched for the period 1995-May 2000 using the strategy below:

#1	mental*
#2	depress* or schizophren*
#3	stress
#4	'eating disorder' or 'eating disorders'
#5	panic or phobia or anxiety
#6	psychiatric or counseling or counselling
#7	psychotherap*
#8	psychiatrist*
#9	#1 or #2 or #3 or #4 or #5 or #6 or #7 or #8

A5.7 The Internet

The Internet will be searched for relevant economic evaluations. Particular emphasis will be put on searching the web sites of organisations indexed in 'Netting the Evidence. A ScHARR Introduction to Evidence Based Practice on the Internet' (http://www.shef.ac.uk/~scharr/ir/netting.html)

APPENDIX 6. DATA EXTRACTION TABLES FOR COST-EFFECTIVENESS PAPERS

Study details	Participants	Intervention	Outcomes	Results	Authors' conclusions	CRD conclusions and implications
Authors Beecham et al, 1996[63] **Source of effectiveness data** Single prospective cohort study **Country** Northern Ireland	Former long-stay psychiatric hospital patients in Northern Ireland	Community care compared with hospital care. The focus was on people who moved from hospital to community accommodation. No specific approaches such as ACT were considered.	Daily living skills, behaviour problems, morale and life satisfaction both pre- and post-discharge into the community	**Effectiveness results** No significant results around mean scale scores were found between hospital and community-based interviews. No significant differences were found between the mean hospital and community-based scores around morale, life satisfaction, and Psychosocial Functioning Inventory subscale scoring. A small significant improvement was discovered post-discharge around the Depression Inventory subscale score (p <0.05). **Cost results** The average weekly cost of providing hospital care for the subject group was found to be £562.82 (range: £443.30 - 674.91) between the 6 hospitals concerned. In comparison, the average weekly cost of providing community care was found to be £295 (range: £234.00 -397.84) between patients discharged from the 6 hospitals concerned. **Synthesis of costs and benefits** No synthesis of costs and benefits was performed	The community care provided to former long-stay psychiatric patients was found to be a cost-effective alternative and no real change in clients' welfare was found in the study, with community care being provided at a far lower cost than its comparator.	The selection of community care and hospital care was justified. Direct costings were well sourced, detailed and analysed with reference to (inflated) price years, although these estimates are reflective of services provided in Northern Ireland alone. No sensitivity analysis, cost conversion(s) or power calculations were provided. This was a well researched and detailed paper although the conclusions regarding the superiority of community-based over hospital-based care would have been strengthened by analysis around economic benefits, resulting cost-effectiveness synthesis of these benefits, and cost savings. **Implications of the study** No implications are reported
Authors Chiverton et al, 1999[64] **Source of effectiveness data** Single RCT **Country** USA	Psychiatric inpatients	Case management services compared with traditional care	Three month follow-up of mental health status, service satisfaction, hospital days and average length of stay.	**Effectiveness results** Intervention group was significantly less depressed after hospital discharge. The intervention group spent fewer days in hospital (181 vs 408 days), with an average length of stay of 20.1 (vs 25.5 in the control group). The two groups reported similar levels of health service satisfaction (based on 27% return rate). **Cost results** The intervention saved $175,375 over the period of analysis. **Synthesis of Cost and benefits** Transitional case management reduced costs while maintaining quality	Transitional case management services maintained quality and reduced costs with a high level of consumer satisfaction.	Results are not generalisable because of limitations in the cost analysis. A more complete economic analysis, including tangible economic outcomes, cost-effectiveness ratios, sensitivity analysis, price years for the treatment regimens would offer more validity in the determination of cost-effectiveness of transitional case management versus traditional care for psychiatric inpatients. **Implications of the study** No implications were reported

Study details	Participants	Intervention	Outcomes	Results	Authors' conclusions	CRD conclusions and implications
Authors Clark et al, 1998[65] **Source of effectiveness data** Single RCT **Country** USA	People with co-occurring severe mental illness and substance use disorders	Assertive Community Treatment (ACT) compared with Standard Case Management (SCM)	Subjective quality of life ratings and substance abuse treatment scale scores.	**Effectiveness results** Participants in both groups experienced significant reductions in their substance use. SCM quality of life increased from 0.61 to 0.65, while ACT quality of life increased from 0.56 to 0.66. Longitudinal analysis showed that SCM was more efficient over the first two years, while ACT was significantly more efficient during the third year. **Cost results** The three year mean total study costs per patient were $ 124,145 (SCM) and $ 118,078 (ACT). ACT and SCM were not significantly different in terms of cost-effectiveness over the three-year period. **Synthesis of costs and benefits** No significant difference was found in either costs or effectiveness between ACT and SCM.	ACT is not more cost effective than SCM, however ACT efficiency appears to improve over time.	The estimates of quality of life may not be reliable. Detailed information and analysis around both direct and indirect costing was provided. The authors used a wide range of analytical techniques and discussed their findings and the limitations surrounding them. Generalisability does not appear to have been addressed by the authors. No power calculations were provided. Activity and/or cost information around non-completers was omitted which may have introduced bias into the results. **Implications of the study** Further research is required around the significant difference on costs and effectiveness in the third and final year of analysis, which have not been examined before.
Authors Creed et al, 1997[66] **Source of effectiveness data** Single RCT **Country** UK	Patients with acute psychiatric illness referred for admission	Day hospital or routine inpatient treatment	Clinical symptoms, social functioning, burden on relatives. Direct and indirect costs over 12 months.	**Effectiveness results** Clinical and social outcomes were similar at 6 and 12 months between both groups. Psychiatric symptoms, social behaviour and role performance were significantly reduced (p<0.001) at 6 and 12 months in both groups. Inpatients recovered faster than day patients did and burden on relatives was significantly less in day hospital group at one year. **Cost results** Median direct costs to the hospital were £1923 (95% confidence interval £750 to £3175) per patient less for day hospital treatment than inpatient treatment. Indirect costs were greater for day patients; when these were included, overall day hospital treatment was £2165 cheaper than inpatient treatment (95% CI: £600 to £3543). **Synthesis of costs and benefits** Not stated	Day patient treatment is cheaper for the 30-40% of potential admissions that can be treated in this way (i.e. who are moderately ill). Carers of day hospital inpatients may bear additional costs. Carers of all patients with acute psychiatric illness are often themselves severely distressed at the time of admission, but day hospital treatment leads to fewer burdens on carers in the long term.	This study has not yet been appraised by the NHS-EED team.

Study details	Participants	Intervention	Outcomes	Results	Authors' conclusions	CRD conclusions and implications
Authors Dickey et al, 1997[67] **Source of effectiveness data** Cross-sectional analysis using aggregate data within a single retrospective cohort study, carried out in three regions **Country** USA	Psychiatrically disabled Medicaid beneficiaries, aged 18 to 64, with a diagnosis of schizophrenia and major affective disorder	Public mental health care in three regions: Boston, Central and Western Massachusetts. Western Massachusetts has a developed community care system, while in Central Massachusetts, the primary locus of care is the hospital, with a few local agencies providing community care. In Boston, care is only provided in mental health centres with small inpatient units.	Mental health status	**Effectiveness results** The mean (SD) mental health status score of clients was 54 (21.4) for Boston, 59 (16.7) for Central Massachusetts, and 52.4 (19.2) for Western Massachusetts. **Cost results** The mean (SD) annual total cost of mental care in the three regions was: Boston $14,947 (17,416), Central Massachusetts $24,254 (24,120), and Western Massachusetts $18,712 (20,189). **Synthesis of costs and benefits** Not stated	Western Massachusetts (community-based care) was more cost-effective than the other regions (Boston and Central Massachusetts).	A justification was given for the comparator used. The results of the effectiveness analysis should be interpreted in the light of the study limitations (i.e. small sample size and observational design). Insufficient details of cost estimation were provided. Costs to patients, and other in society, were not included in the analysis. Cost results might have been underestimated because of the small sample size. Cost results may also not be generalisable to other settings or countries. A sensitivity analysis would have been useful to test the robustness of the study results. **Implications of the study** Further studies are needed
Authors Drummond et al, 1991[68] **Source of effectiveness data** Single RCT **Country** Canada	Caregivers living with a relative with moderate or severe dementia	Caregiver support programme compared with conventional community care	Quality-Adjusted life Years (QALYs) and the Caregiver Quality of Life Instrument (CQLI). Direct costs were to the health service: nursing visits, attendant care, MD visits, other paid help, day programmes and overnight institutional respite. Price information related to 1988.	**Effectiveness results** Relative to conventional community care, the improvement in the caregiver group was not statistically significant but was judged clinically important (p value was not significant). **Cost results** Because there was no statistically significant difference in individual item costs between the two groups, a 'conservative' incremental cost was calculated based on the additional annual cost of the CSP: the programme cost/caregiver /annum = Can$1240 (at 1991 prices). **Synthesis of costs and benefits** Outcome and cost duration was 6 months and the inclusion of treatment side-effects was not relevant. Incremental cost per QALY gained for the caregiver support programme with two level respite care was Can$12365 (costs and benefits not discounted).	A 20% difference from baseline in the CQLI favoured the caregiver support group, although this did not reach statistical significance. A comparison of improvement in quality of life with costs implies an incremental cost per quality-adjusted life year gained of Canadian $20,000 for the caregiver support programme, which compares favourably with other health care interventions. Further, larger studies are required to confirm this result.	(This commentary was not written by CRD, but by the authors of the DH Register). 1) The study has small numbers in both intervention and control groups so the true value of caregiver support programme remains uncertain. 2) The hypothesis was driven. 3) There were no health omissions. 4) The sample size was small and hence there was large variance in the CQLI scores. **Implications of the study** No implications are reported

Study details	Participants	Intervention	Outcomes	Results	Authors' conclusions	CRD conclusions and implications
Authors Fontana & Rosenheck, 1997[69] **Source of effectiveness data** Single non-randomised trial with concurrent controls **Country** USA	Veterans of the Vietnam War, with PTSD (Post-Traumatic Stress Disorder)	Long-term specialised inpatient PTSD units, compared with short-stay specialised PTSD units and to non-specialised general psychiatric units	PTSD scores, psychiatric symptom scores, addiction severity Indices, rating for violent behaviour/ thoughts, rating for social involvement and, lastly, the number of days worked over the previous month	**Effectiveness results** Changes in outcomes from admission to the end of the follow-up year were significantly different across the models for 4 of the 9 outcome measures: PTSD, general distress, and alcohol abuse. Generally, veterans in the short-stay PTSD units and the general psychiatric units showed sustained improvement in these areas, while veterans in the long-stay PTSD units showed a return to the levels at the time of admission. **Cost results** The mean per-patient long-stay PTSD unit cost, for the year following admission, was $47,091 (+/- $20,953). The equivalent short-stay PTSD unit cost was $25,809 (+/- $19,614) and the general psychiatric unit cost was $30,676 (+/- $25,881). Analysis of variance showed statistically significant differences between the three groups, but pair-wise comparisons were not reported. **Synthesis of costs and benefits** A formal synthesis of costs and benefits was not performed.	Improvements in the short-stay PTSD units and the general psychiatric units were greater than those observed in the long-stay PTSD units. Long-stay specialised inpatient PTSD units are costly, relative to short-stay specialised evaluation and brief treatment PTSD units and general psychiatric units. Systematic restructuring of Veterans Affairs inpatient PTSD treatment could result in delivery of effective services to a larger number of veterans.	The reason for the choice of the comparators is clear, as they represented current practices in the authors' settings. Although a comprehensive set of outcome measures was used, the lack of comparability between the characteristics of the three groups limits the interpretability of the results. The authors stated that adjustments were made to compensate for this, but did not report which methods were used. The authors noted that although differences between the groups were statistically significant, they were 'more modest clinically'. Although costs were analysed statistically, costs and quantities were not reported separately. This limits the generalisability of the results to other settings. The authors' conclusions are not justified by the study findings. **Implications of the study** No implications are reported

Study details	Participants	Intervention	Outcomes	Results	Authors' conclusions	CRD conclusions and implications
Authors French et al, 1999[70] **Source of effectiveness data** Single cohort study **Country** USA	Homeless mentally ill chemical abusers	A modified therapeutic community compared with standard services ('treatment as usual').	Substance use, criminal activity, HIV-risk behaviour, psychological status, and a prosocial indicator.	**Effectiveness results** Modified therapeutic community subjects reported significantly greater reductions in criminal activity and psychological dysfunction. Both study groups had significant improvements in the outcome domains of HIV risk and substance use. Using multivariate analyses, the authors showed that the modified therapeutic community programme allowed significant improvements to be achieved in non-drug related criminal behaviour, psychological symptoms, and type of employment taken up. **Cost results** The total (average) intervention cost for the modified therapeutic community group was $29,255.00 per individual, per annum compared with $29,638.00 for the standard care group. **Synthesis of costs and benefits** Costs and benefits were not synthesised.	The results of the study showed that when suitably modified, the therapeutic community approach is an effective treatment alternative for homeless mentally ill chemical abusers, with the potential to be highly cost-effective when compared to standard services.	The selection of modified therapeutic community group and 'treatment as usual' group appears to have been justified. The authors acknowledged that some bias may have crept into the analysis especially around baseline admissions, modified therapeutic community and 'treatment as usual' retrieved cases, and retrieved and non-retrieved cases for each group and that this could have affected the study outcomes. There was disparity between the sample sizes used for both clinical outcomes and cost analysis. A summary measure of benefit was not expressed in the study. Adequate costing information was provided for the chosen perspective. Little information was provided around study subject characteristics (age, etc.). Study group allocation was not mentioned for participants, which may have allowed selection bias, although the authors did employ multivariate statistical techniques to try to control for this. No sensitivity analysis was carried out in what appears to have been a cost-outcomes rather than a cost-effectiveness analysis. The authors concluded that the results should be interpreted with some caution. **Implications of the study** As noted by the authors, further full cost-effectiveness analyses are required that would further assess subgroup analyses around differences and compute cost-effectiveness ratios.

Study details	Participants	Intervention	Outcomes	Results	Authors' conclusions	CRD conclusions and implications
Authors Gater et al, 1997[71] **Source of effectiveness data** Single RCT **Country** UK	People with chronic schizophrenia	Multi-disciplinary community team versus hospital setting (control). The approach used (e.g. ACT) not stated. The team aimed to provide a comprehensive range of community-based mental health services.	Patient's current problems and needs	**Effectiveness results** Met needs scores as percentages of meetable need were as follows for the treatment (and control) subjects: psychotic symptoms = 92 (76); underactivity = 80 (22); medication side-effects = 88 (65); neurotic symptoms = 70 (20); physical disorder = 70 (66); behaviour difficulties = 100 (45); distress = 80 (36); daily living skills = 83 (61); use of public amenities and transport = 83 (44); vocational skills = 26 (25); communication skills = 45 (16); managing finances and affairs = 68 (47). **Cost results** Overall health service costs during the study year were: treatment group = £1,406; control group = £1,199. Indirect costs incurred over a 12 month period: treatment group = £4,403; control group = £3,849. **Synthesis of costs and benefits** A synthesis of costs and benefits was not performed. The per capita cost of services received was £245 higher in the treatment group (not significant due to high individual variability).	Multi-disciplinary community-based teams provide better quality care for chronic schizophrenics and distribute resources more effectively than traditional hospital-based services.	The choice of multi-disciplinary community-based and traditional hospital-based mental health teams as comparators was justified. The measures of economic benefit expressed within the study may not be internally valid given that the authors used primary health outcomes and costs to express benefits. As such a cost-consequences study was performed. No power calculations, sensitivity analysis or discounting was performed. As such the robustness of the findings was not tested. **Implications of the study** More comprehensive studies around the care of chronically mentally ill patient are required in order to evaluate the full extent of any benefits that are to be obtained from operating under multi-disciplinary community-based mental health teams. This will require power calculations and valid measures of (economic) benefit in order to validate claims of (cost-) effectiveness.

Study details	Participants	Intervention	Outcomes	Results	Authors' conclusions	CRD conclusions and implications
Authors Goldberg et al, 1996[72] **Source of effectiveness data** Non-randomised trial with concurrent controls **Country** UK	Patients aged between 16 and 65 suffering from new episodes of depression or anxiety disorders. The patients had not had care from mental health services in the year preceding the episode of illness being considered.	Community team based in a primary care service versus hospital service (control group). The community mental health service was set up on a large council estate. The community team consisted of community nurses, a social worker, an occupational therapist, and a clinical psychologist.	Waiting time, quality of notes, continuity of care, range of interventions offered, adequacy and appropriateness of intervention offered, and patient satisfaction.	**Effectiveness results** There were no significant differences between the groups in clinical outcomes, social problems or social disabilities. Non-urgent cases were examined faster in the community service than in the hospital service (13.5 days versus 47.5 days, P <0.01) although the response time for both services was prompt for cases rated as urgent (1.5 days versus 2.5 days). **Cost results** Health services costs for those patients treated in the community group and in the control group were £2,944 and £4,512 respectively. **Synthesis of costs and benefits** There were no significant differences between groups in terms of clinical outcome, but the community service was most likely to offer home assessment and advice to relatives, and was generally preferred by the patients. Total costs for those patients treated in the community group (£2,944) were ess than for the hospital services (£4,512).	Treatment by the community team was more cost-effective than the hospital services.	The reason for the choice of the comparator is clear, as hospital-based service was considered to be the traditional service. The validity of the effectiveness results may be weakened by the lack of randomisation. Resource utilisation was not reported separately from the costs. However, adequate details of methods of cost estimation were given. To explore the robustness of the results, a sensitivity analysis would have been useful. Given the lack of randomisation, sensitivity analysis, and statistical analysis of the costs, the results need to be treated with some caution. **Implications of the study** No implications are presented
Authors Gournay et al, 1995[73] **Source of effectiveness data** Multicentre RCT (six primary care settings) **Country** UK	Patients affected by non-psychotic problems in need of psychiatric interventions	Immediate community psychiatric nurse (CPN) intervention and CPN intervention, delayed for 12 weeks. The control was continuing GP care.	Symptoms and social outcomes. The effectiveness of nurse therapists was measured using the Life Disruption Rating.	**Effectiveness results** Within each of the two treatment groups, patients improved on all measures over time (p <0.001). However, the difference in outcomes between the two groups was not statistically significant. **Cost results** Cost duration was 24 weeks. Saving of resources per patient due to CPN Intervention vs. GP was £193, taking into account the cost of the CPN intervention of £48 per patient. The saving of resources was due to the reduction in the work absences, valued at £267 per patient. **Synthesis of costs and benefits** If the economic analysis is based on both direct and indirect costs, the CPN intervention is the dominant strategy.	The authors concluded that CPN intervention in primary care for less serious mental health problems is an 'expensive luxury', subtracting resources from people with serious and enduring mental health problems.	The authors themselves stressed that the study has limitations in terms of sample size, duration of follow-up and method used. The reliability of the measure of the final outcome used – QALY - depends on the validity of the methods of estimation used. The calculation of the synthesis excluding the indirect costs is debatable, given that the utility of the reduced absence from work was included in the measure for quality of life. **Implications of the study** Further analysis addressed to validate the findings of this study would be useful.

Study details	Participants	Intervention	Outcomes	Results	Authors' conclusions	CRD conclusions and implications
Authors Hawthorne et al, 1999[75] **Source of effectiveness data** Unclear **Country** USA	Adults suffering from a mental illness and receiving residential treatment	Acute care in short-term residential treatment compared with a psychiatric hospital setting	Severity of clients' disturbance and social functioning, length of stay, satisfaction with services	**Effectiveness results** The two groups had similar health outcomes and levels of satisfaction, though the residential group had more severe symptoms on admission. **Cost results** The mean costs for treating patients in the psychiatric hospital was $7,091 more expensive than for treating the residential. **Synthesis of costs and benefits** Costs and benefits were not combined. The results suggest that short-term residential treatment is dominant as it is as effective as hospital-based treatment, and costs less to administer.	Short-term residential treatment is as effective as hospital treatment, while being a more cost-effective option.	The selection of short-term residential treatment and psychiatric hospital treatment settings was justified. Adequate details of cost estimation were provided, although no price year was stated. No sensitivity analysis or power calculations were provided. Study samples were not similar in a number of demographic areas, which limits the validity of comparability and therefore the outcomes assessed. **Implications of the study** Research in this area should contain more robust economic analysis with adequate and comparable sample sizing and randomised subject allocations. Efforts should be directed towards introducing this cost-effective alternative treatment to hospital care.
Authors Hyde et al, 1987[76] **Source of effectiveness data** Single RCT **Country** UK	Long-stay (>6 months) psychiatric patients.	Hospital hostel ward compared with a district general hospital (DGH) psychiatric unit.	Psychological impairment (psychological impairment rating scale, PIRS and present state examination, PSE), social interactions (remedial problem behaviours scale, RPBS) and satisfaction with living conditions.	**Effectiveness results** PIRS and RPBS estimates significantly favoured the hostel ward. There was no difference according to the clinical measures. Use of social facilities and the time spent in socially useful behaviour was greater for the hostel ward group. **Cost results** The main difference in costs is in the hotel costs, which for the DGH represented 44% of total costs as opposed to only 22% for the hostel. Cost duration was 2 years. **Synthesis of costs and benefits** Incremental costs were negative and incremental benefits were positive.	A hard copy of the article could not be obtained from NHS-EED.	(This commentary was not written by CRD, but by the authors of the DH Register.) 1) The sample size is very small. 2) The hypothesis was driven and there was no sensitivity analysis.

Study details	Participants	Intervention	Outcomes	Results	Authors' conclusions	CRD conclusions and implications
Authors Johnston et al, 1998[77] **Source of effectiveness data** Single RCT **Country** Australia	Severely disabled patients with a mental illness.	An assessment of the costs and outcomes of intensive case management versus routine case management for severely disabled patients with a mental illness.	Incidents of employment (paid, voluntary and sheltered), self-harm/ harm to others, accommodation moves, police/legal services contacts, major life events, medication compliance and retention rate.	**Effectiveness results** Primary health outcome results for the intensive group were (routine figures in parenthesis): incidents of employment = 14% (12%) for one or more day; self-harm/harm to others = 23% (28%); accommodation moves = 9% (5%); police/legal services contact = 4% (7%); major life events= 27% (17%); medication compliance = 80% (84%); retention rate = 89% (69%, p <0.01). **Cost results** Average costs were Aus$28,895 (intensive) and Aus$21,150 (routine) for 12 months of care. **Synthesis of costs and benefits** An incremental cost-effectiveness ratio of Aus$27,661 was found in order to treat one more patient in the intensive case management group to make a clinically significant improvement in functioning. Intensive case management led to increased retention rates as well as significantly improving functioning but at a greater cost.	Significantly more patients were retained in the intensive case management strategy. Other (health) outcomes were similar.	The selection of intensive versus routine case management as comparators was justified. The retention rate is not a proper outcome because this rate should be very high to make this study internally valid in the first place. The estimates of benefit used in the economic analysis are likely to be internally valid. Adequate details of costs were provided although the period of their collection (as well as that of outcomes) was unclear. No power calculation was provided nor were any currency conversions. Ethnicity details were also absent from the paper. **Implications of the study** The authors stipulated that future studies should ascertain whether Aus$27,661 per year for one patient to make a clinically significant improvement is a cost-effective use of mental health resources.
Authors Lehman et al, 1999[78] **Source of effectiveness data** Single RCT **Country** USA	152 homeless patients with severe mental illness	Assertive Community Treatment (ACT) or usual services	Followed up for one year to assess stable housing (non institutionalised setting not intended to serve the homeless). Costs included fee-for-service and budgeted services (all ACT costs).	**Effectiveness results** ACT programme was significantly more effective in producing days of stable housing than standard care. **Cost results** ACT programme spent on average $241 in total treatment costs to achieve a day of stable housing compared with $415 for the comparison group, an efficiency ratio of 0.58. **Synthesis of costs and benefits** The incremental cost-effectiveness ratio comparing the two groups was not statistically significant.	ACT provides a cost-effective approach to reducing homelessness among people with severe and persistent mental illness. It is more effective and no more expensive than usual services.	This study has not yet been appraised by the NHS-EED team.

Study details	Participants	Intervention	Outcomes	Results	Authors' conclusions	CRD conclusions and implications
Authors Mangen et al, 1983[79] **Source of effectiveness data** Single RCT **Country** UK	99 psychiatric patients	Community Psychiatric Nurse (CPN) compared with out-patient (OP) care	Followed up for 18 months. Symptom severity, levels of social role performance, degree of family burden. Health service use (contact, admissions, medication use etc.), employment, patient costs.	**Effectiveness results** There were no differences in outcomes between the two groups in symptom severity, levels of social role performance and degree of family burden. Symptom levels and degree of family burden imposed were relatively mild throughout the study period, while there was moderate impairment in the performance of social roles. There was a general tendency for improvement over time in each of these areas. Consumer satisfaction was significantly greater over time among nursing patients. **Cost Results** There was no statistically significant difference in the mean public expenditure for the two models of care. The direct costs of psychiatric care comprised a small proportion of total public expenditure and were initially greater in the nursing group. **Synthesis of costs and benefits** Costs and benefits were not synthesised.	These results confirm the benefit of community psychiatric nursing for this patient group.	This study has not yet been appraised by the NHS-EED team.
Authors McCrone et al, 1994[80] **Source of effectiveness data** Single RCT **Country** UK	Psychotic patients with long term mental health problems	Intensive support provided by a Community Support Team consisting of Community Psychiatric Nurses (CPN) compared with generic or standard care (i.e. routine out-patient consultations and time-limited involvement by CPNs).	Accommodation, employment and income, service use, service costs	**Effectiveness results** The paper reports only service use and cost-effectiveness. **Cost results** The economic evaluation found a cost difference between the groups. Generic group costs averaged £89 per patient per week more than Community Support Team group costs. The difference was only significant for the first 6 months. Changes in the burden of cost across agencies were observed. **Synthesis of costs and benefits** Costs and benefits were not synthesised.	Although CPN inputs and costs were higher for the Community Support Team group, there was a significant short-term reduction in total costs. Beyond the short term, the Community Support Team did not confer costs or cost-effectiveness advantages.	This study has not yet been appraised by the NHS-EED team.

Study details	Participants	Intervention	Outcomes	Results	Authors' conclusions	CRD conclusions and implications
Authors Merson et al, 1996[81] **Source of effectiveness data** Single RCT **Country** UK	Patients with emergency presentation to the psychiatric service via the A&E Department, liaison psychiatrist and approved social worker. Included patients with schizophrenia and related disorders, mood disorder, neurotic and stress-related disorders, substance misuse and personality disorder only.	Community service (Early Intervention Service - EIS) The multidisciplinary EIS team comprised of two community mental health workers, two social workers, a clinical psychologist, an occupational therapist, a senior psychiatrist and an administrator. The comparison was a district general hospital-based psychiatric unit with in-patient and out-patient psychiatric care, day hospital, community psychiatric nursing, clinical pathology and mental health social services.	Ratings of psychopathology and social functioning	**Effectiveness results** Ratings of psychopathology improved significantly in both groups. No significant differences in terms of social functioning between the two groups. **Cost results** The total group cost for the community-based (EIS) and hospital-based (HS) groups were: primary care: £680 (EIS) & £789 (HS) community psychiatric: £24,112 (EIS) &£1,011 (HS) social: £1,075 (EIS) & £2,521 (HS) hospital psychiatric: £13,569 (EIS) & £110,065 (HS) general hospital: £8,218 (EIS) and £8,818 (HS) custodial: £2,416 (EIS) and £3,536 (HS) miscellaneous services: £5,631 (EIS) and £3,360 (HS) . The respective total costs for each group were £35,701 and £130,100. Both the total cost and average cost per patient was considerably less for the community service than for the hospital service. Duration of costs was three months. **Synthesis of costs and benefits** Costs and benefits were not synthesised.	Taken together with clinical outcome, which showed no advantages for the hospital-based service over the community-based service, our findings suggest that this form of community psychiatric service is a cost-efficient alternative to hospital-based care for this group of patients.	The study design used was appropriate to answer the question posed with good internal and external validity. **Implications of the study** No implications are reported
Authors Morriss et al, 1998[82] **Source of effectiveness data** Prospective before-and-after study. **Country** UK	Patients presenting at GP surgeries with somatised mental disorders (medically unexplained symptoms)	GP training package to encourage patients with somatised mental disorders to reattribute and relate physical symptoms to psychosocial problems.	Successfully treated patients using a self-rated psychiatric symptom questionnaire (GHQ-12). Direct costs included GP practice visits, drugs, hospital costs, GP training.	**Effectiveness results** At 1 month after training the cohort effectively treated 2% more patients than before-training, and 17% more patients at 3 months. **Cost results** Total costs for pre-training were £ 34,134 and £28,912 for post-training. The average cost effectiveness was £ 1034 pre-training and £ 578 post-training, resulting in a marginal cost-effectiveness ratio of £324,83. **Synthesis of costs and benefits** Costs and benefits were not synthesised.	Training GPs with the reattribution training package appears to be extremely cost-effective. However, the results should be interpreted with caution.	Disparity between sample sizes used for both clinical outcomes and clinical analysis. Summary measure of benefit was not expressed in the study. Adequate cost information was provided for the chosen perspective. Study group allocation was not mentioned, although multivariate statistical techniques used to try and control for this. No sensitivity analyses were carried out May be a cost-outcomes rather than a cost-effectiveness analysis. **Implications of the study** No implications are reported

Study details	Participants	Intervention	Outcomes	Results	Authors' conclusions	CRD conclusions and implications
Authors Smith et al, 1995[83] **Source of effectiveness data** Single RCT **Country** USA	Patients with a history of somatisation disorders or 6-12 years of unexplained medical symptoms	Guidelines for primary care physicians of patients with somatisation problems compared with no guidelines. Guidelines consisted of information about the condition, suggesting regular appointments and physical examination.	Self-reported general health status, social functioning, mental health and physical functioning	**Effectiveness results** Patients of physicians who received the intervention reported significantly increased physical functioning that remained stable during the year after the intervention. **Cost results** The intervention reduced annual medical charges by $289 in 1990 constant dollars, a 32.9% reduction in annual median charges for medical care. This reduction remained stable at 2 years after the intervention. **Synthesis of costs and benefits** The use of guidelines for somatisation disorders is an effective and cost-effective intervention, as it reduces subsequent charges for medical care, while improving health outcomes.	The present study describes a successful test of a psychiatric consultation intervention for patients who somatised but who did not meet diagnostic criteria for somatisation disorders.	Cluster randomised trial, with unit of allocation different from unit of analysis. Proper analysis should take into account the fact that randomisation was at the physician, not the patient level. The most likely result is that the precision of the effectiveness data was exaggerated. Charge data were used to approximate costs and patient costs were not accounted for within the study. **Implications of the study** Guidelines should be provided to physicians, reducing the incidence of unnecessary diagnostic procedures and treatment. Further research is required to see whether results can be generalised to other populations.
Authors Tyrer et al, 1998[84] **Source of effectiveness data** Multicentre RCT (two sites) **Country** UK	Patients aged 16 to 65 years with severe mental illness (psychosis or severe non-psychosis mood disorder), with a previous admission within the past 3 years	Community multidisciplinary teams compared to hospital-based care programmes, after discharge from inpatient care. Both intervention and control used a care programme approach.	Rates of clinical psychopathology depression, anxiety and social functioning.	**Effectiveness results** The clinical outcomes were similar for both community care and hospital care. **Cost results** The hospital and community group costs were £1,165,676 and £1,286,628, respectively. The average cost was £16,765 for the community group versus £19,125 for the hospital group. Costs of the hospital-based care group "were 14% greater per patient than in the community group. This was dwarfed by a twofold difference in the costs of care in the outer London services compared with those in the inner London services". **Synthesis of costs and benefits** The estimated benefits and costs were not combined, since aftercare by community teams had a similar outcome with less costs.	Delivery of care by community-based teams offers no advantage in terms of clinical outcome over equivalent hospital-based teams. The hospital care programme was more expensive.	The reason for the choice of comparator is clear. The comparator chosen (hospital-based care programmes) was commonly used for patients with severe mental illness. Random assignment of patients to the two models of care, decreases the possibility of bias. However there is no evidence of adjustment for confounding variables. More details about the methods of quantity/cost estimation would have been useful as would information about the sources of the quantity and cost data. A sensitivity analysis was not carried out, therefore the results may not be generalisable to other settings. **Implications of the study** No implications are reported

Study details	Participants	Intervention	Outcomes	Results	Authors' conclusions	CRD conclusions and implications
Authors UK700 case management trial 2000[74] **Source of effectiveness data** Multicentre RCT **Country** UK	708 patients with psychosis and a history of repeated hospital admissions	Intensive case management (case loads 10-15) compared with standard case management (case-loads 30-35)	Days in hospital for psychiatric problems over 24 months, clinical status, quality of life, social disability and patient satisfaction.	**Effectiveness results** There was no significant difference between the two groups in days in hospital, clinical outcomes, quality of life, social disability or patient satisfaction scores. **Cost results** No significant differences were found in the average overall costs for care per patient between the intensive and standard case management. The observed cost per patient (£1849) appears to be accounted mainly by the difference in the cost of case management per patient (£1830), with little impact of intensive case management being observed in the non-health care sectors. No statistically significant differences were found between the two interventions. Case management constituted 13% of the total cost of care of the intensive group and 6% of the standard group. Staffed accommodation also made a relatively large contribution to the total costs of care. **Synthesis of costs and benefits** Since the two forms of case management did not differ in effectiveness or cost, a formal cost effectiveness analysis was not needed. Psychiatric in-patient costs comprised almost half of the total costs of care for the patients in both the standard (48%) and intensive groups (47%).	Reduced case-loads have no clear beneficial effects on costs, clinical outcome or cost-effectiveness. The policy of advocating intensive case management for patients with severe psychosis is not supported by these results.	This study has not yet been appraised by the NHS-EED team

Study details	Participants	Intervention	Outcomes	Results	Authors' conclusions	CRD conclusions and implications
Authors Van Minnen et al, 1997[85] **Source of effectiveness data** Single RCT **Country** The Netherlands	Patients with mild, or borderline, mental retardation	Specialised hospital treatment compared with outreach treatment	Psychiatric symptoms measured by four rating scales.	**Effectiveness results** The two groups showed no significant differences with regards to psychiatric symptoms. The burden of carers was similar for both outreach treatment group and hospital treatment group. Admission to the hospital could be limited for 84% of the outreach-treated patients. **Cost results** The mean total cost per patient for the hospital group was $41,134 and for the outreach treatment group was $24,221. Outreach treatment costs were 40% lower than hospital treatment costs. **Synthesis of costs and benefits** Not applicable. Outreach treatment represents an effective and efficient alternative to hospital treatment for patients with mental retardation and psychiatric disorders.	Outreach treatment represents an effective alternative to hospital treatment for patients with mental retardation and psychiatric disorders. The authors concluded that there were no differences in the primary health outcomes, and hence, the economic analysis was based on costs only.	The number of subjects was small and the power to establish equivalence with 90% confidence intervals exceeded 0.80 for only one of the four outcome measures used. The resource quantities were not reported separately from the costs. No adequate details were reported of the method of quantity/cost estimation. The costs included for the hospital treatment group should have been reported. The hospitalisation costs of patients in the outreach treatment group were not included. Also, the "hotel costs" for treatment in alternative modes of accommodation (e.g. group homes) were not included, and therefore it would have been appropriate to separate this item from the cost of hospital treatment. The authors' conclusions may not be fully justified. The conclusions regarding equivalence may not be justified due to an inadequate sample size, and the validity of the cost comparison clearly needs further clarification. Due to the lack of detail regarding resources and prices the generalisability of the result to other setting cannot be assessed.

Study details	Participants	Intervention	Outcomes	Results	Authors' conclusions	CRD conclusions and implications
Authors Von Korff et al, 1998[86] **Source of effectiveness data** Two RCTs **Country** USA	Subjects suffering from depressive illness	Collaborative care in the primary setting (patients co-managed by the primary care physician and a consultant psychiatrist or psychologist). The control was usual care.	Proportions of successfully treated patients in the major depression group and the minor depression group. A successfully treated patient was defined as a 50% or greater reduction in SCL-90 depression symptom score at the 4-month follow-up.	**Effectiveness results** For psychiatrist consultation services the proportions successfully treated for major depression was 0.744 (intervention) and 0.438 (control); and for minor depression was 0.6 (intervention) and 0.679 (control). For psychologist interventions with brief therapy the proportions successfully treated for major depression were 0.704 (intervention) and 0.423 (control), and 0.667 and 0.528 respectively for minor depression. **Cost results** The cost per patient treated in the psychiatrist consultation services for major depression was $1,337 (intervention) and $850 (control) and for minor depression was $1,298 (intervention) and $656 (control). The cost per patient treated in the psychologist intervention with brief therapy for major depression was $1,182 (intervention) and $918 (control) and for minor depression was $1,045 and $525 respectively. **Synthesis of costs and benefits** Incremental cost-effectiveness was computed for: (1) psychiatrist consultation services, collaborative management; major depression $1,592 and minor depression -$8,190. (2) psychologist intervention with brief therapy, collaborative management; major depression $940 and minor depression $3,741.	Collaborative care increased depression treatment costs and improved the cost-effectiveness of treatment for patients with major depression	The selection of usual care and collaborative care as comparators was justified. Benefits were expressed in terms of proportions of successfully treated patients and success was assessed by a reliable method. Sample sizes were small and no statistical analyses of health benefits were undertaken. As such the results need to be treated with a degree of caution. Cost estimates appear to be valid although no (common) price year was stated. A comprehensive list of cost items was provided. Indirect costs were not assessed which might be relevant for those patients who were in employment. Withdrawal data were not included in the final analysis of costs and cost-effectiveness. Small samples were used in compilation of average costings for both papers and for both minor and major depression. **Implications of the study** The results suggest that, by targeting patients with major depression in the primary care setting, effective treatment can be achieved with only modest increases in the cost of treating depression. Redeployment of some mental health professionals from the speciality setting to primary care clinics may result in a more cost-effective use of their skills. The results need to be validated, however, by large-scale randomised controlled trials.

Study details	Participants	Intervention	Outcomes	Results	Authors' conclusions	CRD conclusions and implications
Authors Wiersma et al, 1995[87] **Source of effectiveness data** Single RCT **Country** The Netherlands	Patients with affective and schizophrenic disorders	Day treatment compared with hospital treatment	Present State Examination (PSE) scores, compliance, number of patient contacts, social functioning, and satisfaction with care	**Effectiveness results** Patients in the day treatment (experimental) group showed greater compliance and longer episodes of treatment. Experimental subjects also had twice as many contacts as controls during the two years (41.3 vs 22.3 contacts for affective patients and 39.7 vs 20.5 contacts for schizophrenic patients; p=0.024). There were no differences between the two groups in the course of psychopathology. However, significant improvement was found among experimental subjects in self-care. Experimental group patients and their families were significantly more satisfied with the treatment. Health benefits were not discounted. **Cost results** The costs were not clearly stated. It was mentioned however, that the extra cost of community care was less than 2%. It was not stated whether costs were discounted. **Synthesis of costs and benefits** Day treatment with community care led to a significant health benefits compared with conventional hospital care in terms of compliance, social functioning, and satisfaction with care, although at a slightly higher cost. Day treatment with community care was a cost-effective alternative to standard clinical care.	Day treatment leads to a higher number of contacts with the ambulatory service, and therefore to greater continuity of care with prolonged episodes of treatment. This indicates greater compliance and less discharge against medical advice, but also greater dependency on mental health care. The course of psychopathology does not differ significantly but day treatment results in better social functioning and higher satisfaction with care.	This study suffers from major problems with the analysis of costs. The authors claimed that there was no statistical difference between the two treatment types in total costs as both treatment types were reimbursed in the same way (in order to render the experiment financially neutral and acceptable to the hospital). This approach, however, ignored the fact that, reimbursement aside, costs could differ between the two treatment types. Some comparison between the structure of costs was made, but many important costs, such as the extra costs for patients and their families, were not observed. Cost results therefore remain assumptions and this study is hypothesis generating. **Implications of the study** By providing evidence on the effectiveness of day treatment with community care, this study raises issues around the establishment of day treatment facilities, community care, and rehabilitation programmes.

Study details	Participants	Intervention	Outcomes	Results	Authors' conclusions	CRD conclusions and implications
Authors Weisbrod et al, 1980[88] **Source of effectiveness data** Single centre, prospective controlled trial **Country** USA	Persons with mental disorders	Community-based alternative to mental hospital treatment called "Training in Community Living" (TCL) compared with traditional hospital-based treatment	Clinical symptomatology, employment status, family burden, patient satisfaction with life, illegal activity, hospital costs	**Effectiveness results** The community group were significantly less symptomatic on 7 of 13 measures; on the other 6, no significant differences were found. Patient satisfaction with life was also significantly higher for the community group. **Cost results** Total costs were: more than £7,200 per patient per year for both programmes. Very sizeable proportions of the costs (between 40 and 50%) are in forms other than direct costs for either treatment. Considering all forms of costs in total the hospital-based programme is about 10% cheaper per patient. **Synthesis of costs and benefits** Experimental program provided additional benefits and costs as compared with control. However the added benefits, $1,200 per patient per year, are nearly $400 more per patient than added costs.	The community programme is cost saving from a societal viewpoint but more costly to the health service. A number of the forms of benefits and costs that we have measured in qualitative but nonmonetary terms show additional advantages of the community-based experimental program. The generalisability of a single experiment is limited, but the methodologies developed may be useful if their proper role is appreciated.	None reported
Authors Wolff et al, 1997[89] **Source of effectiveness data** Single RCT **Country** USA	Mentally ill people who are homeless or at risk of homelessness	Patients were randomised to one of three interventions: Assertive Community Treatment (ACT) alone, ACT with community workers (CW) who was assigned to each client, and brokered Case Management (CM)	Psychiatric symptoms (Brief Psychiatric Rating Scale), days in stable housing, client satisfaction, and program contact. Service use and costs.	**Effectiveness results** Compared to the CM group, clients in the two ACT groups had fewer symptoms at 18 months, reported more contact with their case managers ($p<0.05$), and were more satisfied with their treatment programmes ($p<0.01$).There was no significant effect on stable housing at 18 months. **Cost results** Total cost over 18-month study for average client in ACT alone was $49,510, ACT + CW $39,913 and CM $45,076. No significant differences between groups in total costs over 18 months. Major differences in the percentage of costs associated with each cost category, especially in first 6 months. Average cost for inpatient services decreased by $1,315 for ACT + CW, increased by $4,484 for ACT and increased by $ 8,973 for CM. **Synthesis of costs and benefits** Not stated	ACT is more cost-effective than brokered CM for people with mental illness. However, this finding should be treated with caution, as only 85 of the 165 participants provided data for the cost-effectiveness study.	This study has not yet been appraised by the NHS-EED team.